Visit our website

to find out about other books and our sister companies in H...

Register free at
www.harcourt-international...

and you will get

- the latest information on new books, journals and electronic products in your chosen subject areas

- the choice of e-mail or post alerts or both, when there are any new books in your chosen areas

- news of special offers and promotions

- information about products from all Harcourt Health Sciences companies including Baillière Tindall, Churchill Livingstone, Mosby and W. B. Saunders

You will also find an easily searchable catalogue, online ordering, information on our extensive list of journals...and much more!

Visit the Harcourt Health Sciences website today!

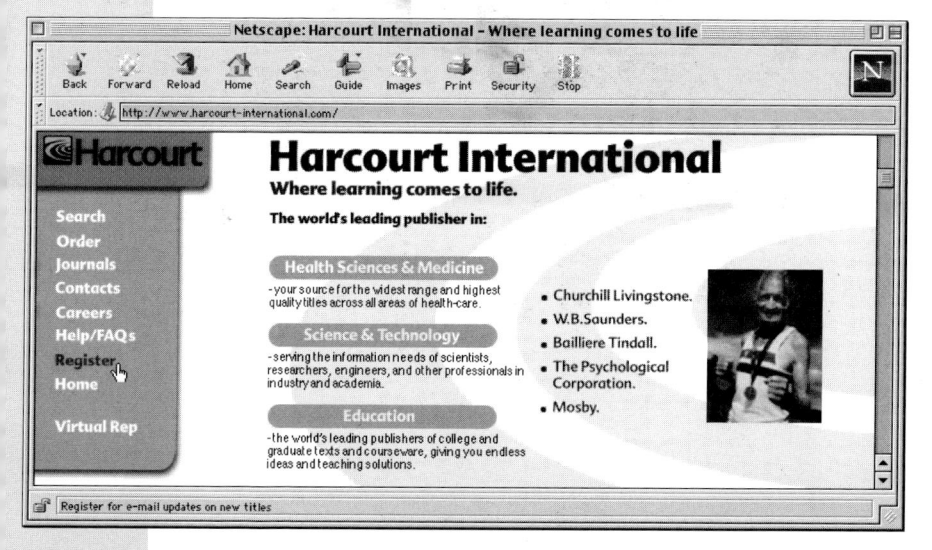

Harcourt Health Sciences

COMPLETE DATA INTERPRETATION FOR THE MRCP

Commissioning Editor: Laurence Hunter
Project Manager: Fiona Conn
Designer: Erik Bigland

COMPLETE DATA INTERPRETATION FOR THE MRCP

Steve Hughes MRCP

Senior Registrar in Geriatrics and General Internal Medicine,
St. George's Hospital Medical School, London

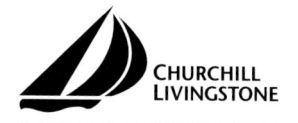

CHURCHILL
LIVINGSTONE

EDINBURGH LONDON NEW YORK PHILADELPHIA ST LOUIS SYDNEY
TORONTO 2001

CHURCHILL LIVINGSTONE

An imprint of Harcourt Publishers Limited

© Harcourt Publishers Limited 2001

D is a registered trademark of Harcourt Publishers Limited

The right of Steven Hughes to be identified as author of this work has been asserted by him in accordance with the Copyright, Designs and Patents Act 1988

All rights reserved. No part of this publication may be reproduced, stored in a retrieval system, or transmitted in any form or by any means, electronic, mechanical, photocopying, recording or otherwise, without either the prior permission of the publishers (Harcourt Publishers Limited, Harcourt Place, 32 Jamestown Road, London NW1 7BY), or a licence permitting restricted copying in the United Kingdom issued by the Copyright Licensing Agency, 90 Tottenham Court Road, London W1P 0LP.

First published 2001

ISBN 0443064466

British Library Cataloguing in Publication Data
A catalogue record for this book is available from the British Library

Library of Congress Cataloging in Publication Data
A catalog record for this book is available from the Library of Congress

Note
Medical knowledge is constantly changing. As new information becomes available, changes in treatment, procedures, equipment and the use of drugs become necessary. The author and the publishers have taken care to ensure that the information given in this text is accurate and up-to-date. However, readers are strongly advised to confirm that the information, especially with regard to drug usage, complies with the latest legislation and standards of practice.

The publisher's policy is to use **paper manufactured from sustainable forests**

Printed in China

PREFACE

There are many books available which, like this one, are aimed at candidates for the MRCP Part 2 Exam. However, in contrast to other MRCP revision aids, which provide only one or two examples of diseases that can be diagnosed by a particular test or investigation, this book aims to cover, for each investigation, all of the outcomes that one might expect to come up in the exam.

Part 1 consists of the questions and these are ordered by system for easy reference. Part 2 comprises the answers to the questions and is also ordered by system. In addition to an overview of each investigation, this section is heavily illustrated with annotated diagrams, tables of 'causes', clinical pointers and comprehensive revision notes, allowing the book to serve as both a reference text and a revision aid. I hope you find it useful.

S.H. 2000

NORMAL VALUES

Haematology

Haemoglobin (Hb)	– Male	13.5–17.5 g/dL
	– Female	11.5–15.5 g/dL
Red cell count (RCC)	– Male	4.5–6.5×10^{12}/L
	– Female	3.9–5.6×10^{12}/L
White cell count (WCC)		4.0–11.0×10^{9}/L
Neutrophils		40–75%
Lymphocytes		20–45%
Monocytes		2–10%
Basophils		0–1%
Eosinophils		1–6%
Platelets		550×10^{9}/L
Reticulocytes		< 2%
MCH		27–32 pg
MCHC		31–35 g/dL
PCV		0.40–0.54
MCV		76–98 fL
RDW		13.2 ± 1.6%
HbA_2		normal < 3.5%
ESR	– Male	Half age
	– Female	Half (age + 10)

Biochemistry

Sodium	136–149 mmol/L
Potassium	3.8–5.0 mmol/L
Urea	2.5–6.5 mmol/L
Creatinine	55–110 µmol/L
Calcium (total)	2.1–2.6 mmol/L
Phosphate	0.80–1.40 mmol/L
Magnesium	0.75–1.05 mmol/L
Fasting blood glucose	
– Normal	< 6.0 mmol/L
– Impaired fasting glucose tolerance	6.1–6.9 mmol/L
– Diabetes	> 7.0 mmol/L
Chloride	95–105 mmol/L
Uric acid	180–420 µmol/L
Total protein	65–80 g/L
Albumin	35–55 g/L
IgA	0.8–4.0 g/L

IgG	5.3–16.5 g/L
IgM	0.5–2.0 g/L
Bilirubin	< 17 µmol/L
AST	13–42 IU/L
ALP – Adults	40–115 U/L
– Before puberty	< 400 U/L
Gamma GT	< 40 IU/L
CK	70–175 IU/L
LDH	100–300 IU/L
Caeruloplasmin	200–400 mg/L
Ferritin	< 300 µg/L
Transferrin saturation	< 60%
Serum B_{12}	200–900 pg/ml
Red cell folate	0.36–1.44 µmol/L
Fibrinogen	2.0–4.0 g/L
CRP	< 10 mg/L
Plasma osmolarity	278–305 mOsm/kg

Endocrinology

Total T4		70–140 nmol/L
Free T4		9.0–22.0 pmol/L
Total T3		1.2–3.0 nmol/L
Free T3		2.9–8.9 pmol/L
TSH		0.5–5.7 mU/L
Prolactin		< 600 U/L
Cortisol	Midnight	170–260 nmol/L
	9 am	170–770 nmol/L

Stool

Faecal fat	< 18 mmol/24 hours

Urine

Urine osmolarity	60–1500 mOsm/kg
Urinary sodium	100–250 mmol/24 hours
Urinary potassium	14–120 mmol/24 hours

Arterial Blood Gases

pH	7.35–7.45
paO_2	> 10.6 kPa
$paCO_2$	4.7–6.0 kPa
Bicarbonate	24–30 mmol/L
Base excess	± 2 mmol/L

PICTURE ACKNOWLEDGEMENTS

Fig. 1.13 reproduced with permission from A. J. Camm 'Cardiovascular Disease' in P. J. Kumar and M. L. Clark, eds. 'Clinical Medicine', 2nd edition (Baillière Tindall, 1990), p. 538

Fig. 1.36 reproduced with permission from D. J. Pennell and E. Prvulovich 'Nuclear Cardiology' (British Nuclear Society, 1995), p. 58

CONTENTS

Investigations checklist xii

Part 1: Questions

1. Cardiology 2
2. Endocrinology 24
3. Haematology 38
4. Renal medicine 51
5. Rheumatology 64
6. Neurology 72
7. Respiratory medicine 84
8. Gastroenterology 93

Part 2: Answers

1. Cardiology 102
2. Endocrinology 135
3. Haematology 175
4. Renal medicine 195
5. Rheumatology 215
6. Neurology 234
7. Respiratory medicine 249
8. Gastroenterology 263

INVESTIGATIONS CHECKLIST

Please note: In addition to the specific investigations detailed below, all sections contain questions involving interpretation of general biochemistry and haematology data.

	Question Number
Cardiology	
Cardiac Catheter Studies	1.1–1.7, 1.46, 2.23
Electrocardiogram	1.8–1.17, 1.23
Echocardiography	1.18–1.22
Radionuclide Imaging	1.23
Endocrinology	
Dexamethasone Suppression Test	2.2–2.4
Synacthen Test	2.6
Thyroid Function Tests	2.7–2.12
Sex Hormones	2.13–2.15, 2.18
Glucose Tolerance Test	2.17, 2.24
Haematology	
Coagulation Tests	3.6–3.9, 3.13–3.15
Bone Marrow Cytochemistry	3.10
Paul–Bunnel Test	3.11
Blood Film Results	3.5, 3.13–3.16, 3.19, 3.22, 8.4
Coombe's Test	3.15
Haematinics	3.20, 8.1, 8.4
Renal	
Renal Biopsy Results	4.1
Urine Biochemistry	2.16, 4.1–4.2
Urine Microscopy	4.4, 5.1
Isotope Renography	4.6
Water Deprivation Test	4.8–4.10
Plasma/Urine Osmolality	4.2, 4.7–4.12
Acid-base Balance	4.13–4.15, 4.17–4.21
Rheumatology	
Autoantibody Tests	5.1, 5.3, 5.5–5.8, 5.11, 5.12, 6.8, 8.10
Complement	4.4, 5.2
Immunoglobulins	5.2, 8.8, 8.9
ANCA	5.3, 5.6, 5.11, 6.8
Synovial Fluid Examination	5.9–5.12

Neurology

CSF Examination (Lumbar Puncture)	6.1–6.6
EEG	6.4–6.6
EMG	6.7, 6.8
Visual Evoked Potentials (VEP)	6.9
Nerve Conduction Studies	6.10, 6.11
Audiology	6.12–6.16

Respiratory

Spirometry	7.1, 7.3, 7.5–7.7, 7.9, 7.11, 7.13
Flow Volume Curves	7.2, 7.4, 7.8, 7.10, 7.12
Arterial Blood Gases	4.13–4.15, 4.17, 4.18, 4.21
Diffusion Studies	7.3, 7.5, 7.7, 7.9, 7.11, 7.13

Gastroenterology

Gut Hormones	2.22, 2.23
D-Xylose Absorption Test	8.2
Schilling Test	8.6
Liver Biopsy Results	8.8
Jejunal Biopsy Results	8.10

PART 1

QUESTIONS

Answers on page

A → 101

1 CARDIOLOGY

CARDIOLOGY

1.1

These are the pressure and saturation data from a cardiac catheter study performed on a 20-year-old woman. The catheter study was necessary because of the findings from an echocardiogram that had been requested for investigation of a systolic murmur.

	Pressure (mm Hg)	Saturation (%)
SVC	–	67
RA (mean)	8	80
RV	27/1	79
PA	25/8	81
LA (mean)	8	98
LV	115/0	96
Aorta	110/70	97

a) What is the most likely diagnosis?
b) What complications may occur in this condition?
c) What two abnormalities might be seen on ECG?
d) What is the recommended treatment?

A → 103

1.2

Below are the results of a cardiac catheter study performed on a 45-year-old male with blackouts, a heaving apex beat and a murmur.

	Pressure (mm Hg)	Saturation (%)
RA (mean)	5	77
RV	30/7	76
PA	30/12	77
LV	192/8	95
Femoral artery	150/82	93

a) What is the most likely diagnosis?
b) What further information do you require from the catheter study?
c) What treatment should be given?

A → 104

1.3

These are the results of a cardiac catheter study performed on an 18-year-old girl who complained of increased shortness of breath on exertion.

	Pressure (mmHg)	Saturation (%)
RA (mean)	8	77
RV	–	84
PA	53/18	85
PCWP (mean)	18	–
LV	98/10	96
Aorta	100/70	97

a) What is the most likely diagnosis?
b) What is the most appropriate treatment?

A → 105

1.4

Here are the results of a cardiac catheter study performed on a 55-year-old woman for investigation of severe shortness of breath on exertion, orthopnoea and paroxysmal nocturnal dyspnoea.

	Pressure (mmHg)	Saturation (%)
RA (mean)	13	75
RV	85/0–13	74
PA	82/44	–
LA (mean)	22	93
LV	118/0–4	93
Aorta	115/60	91

a) What is the most likely diagnosis and what is the most likely cause?
b) What complication has arisen?
c) What other complications can occur?
d) Is conservative treatment appropriate?

A → 106

CARDIOLOGY

1.5

These are the results from a cardiac catheter study performed on a 26-year-old woman who was being investigated for palpitations.

	Pressure (mmHg)	Saturation (%)
RA (mean)	8	83
RV	29/0	82
PA	29/13	–
LA (mean)	11	95
LV	115/0	–
Aorta	110/70	95
Femoral vein	–	73

a) What is the most likely diagnosis?
b) Below are the results of a catheter study performed 10 years later. What complication has developed?

A → 106

	Pressure (mmHg)	Saturation (%)
RA (mean)	17	68
RV	–	67
PA	75/25	67
PCWP (mean)	14	87
LV	98/10	86
Aorta	100/70	87

1.6

A cardiac catheter study was performed on an 18-month-old infant with cyanosis and failure to thrive. The results are shown below.

	Pressure (mmHg)	Saturation (%)
SVC	–	51
RA (mean)	10	50
RV	110/8	50
PA	15/6	51
LA (mean)	13	98
LV	110/10	84
Aorta	110/80	77

a) What cardiac abnormalities are present (name three)?
b) What is the most likely diagnosis?
c) What is the expected appearance of the lung fields on plain X-ray?

A → 107

5

1.7

A 35-year-old woman is admitted with a two-week history of high fever and general malaise. A characteristic murmur is heard on clinical examination and echocardiography reveals a hypertrophied but dilated left ventricle and a dilated left atrium. The results of subsequent cardiac catheterization are shown below.

	Pressure (mmHg)	Saturation (%)
RA (mean)	8	75
RV	–	76
PA	50/17	86
PCWP (mean)	16	–
LV	140/10	96
Aorta	140/50	97

a) What diagnosis is indicated from the catheter study?
b) What complications have developed (name two)?
c) Describe the characteristic murmur.

A → 108

CARDIOLOGY

1.8

A 21-year-old man presented to the Accident and Emergency department feeling light-headed. This settled following intravenous injection of a drug and the subsequent ECG is shown below.

a) What is the diagnosis?
b) What drug was given?

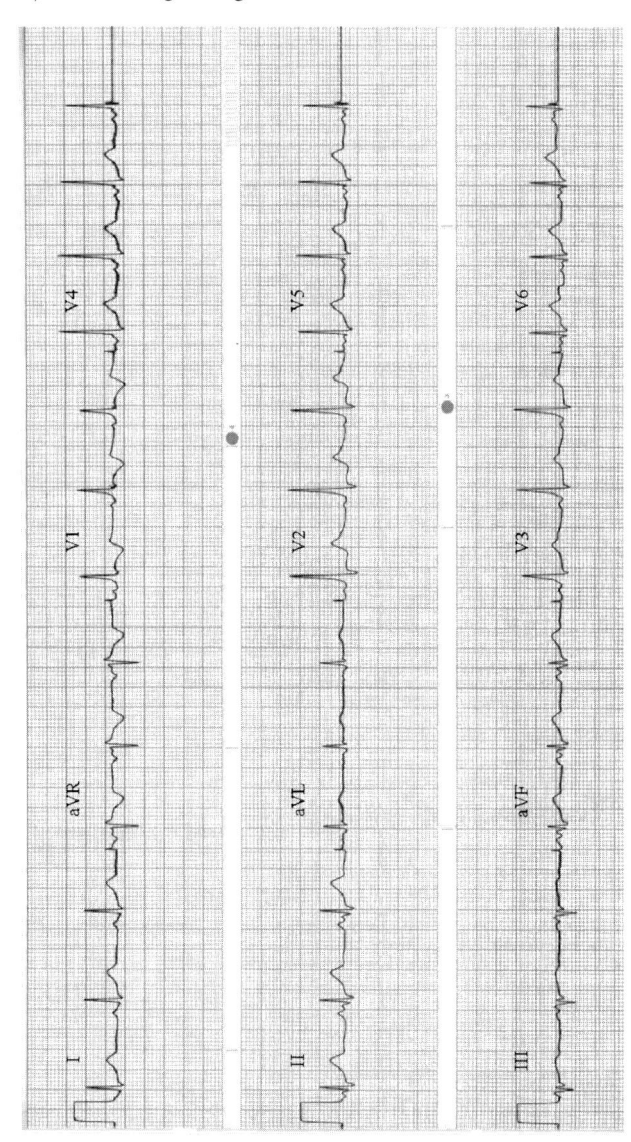

A → 109

Fig. 1.1

1.9

Below is the ECG of a 61-year-old publican who has presented with sudden-onset dizziness and shortness of breath.

a) What is the diagnosis?
b) Name three possible causes.
c) What treatment is indicated?

A → 111

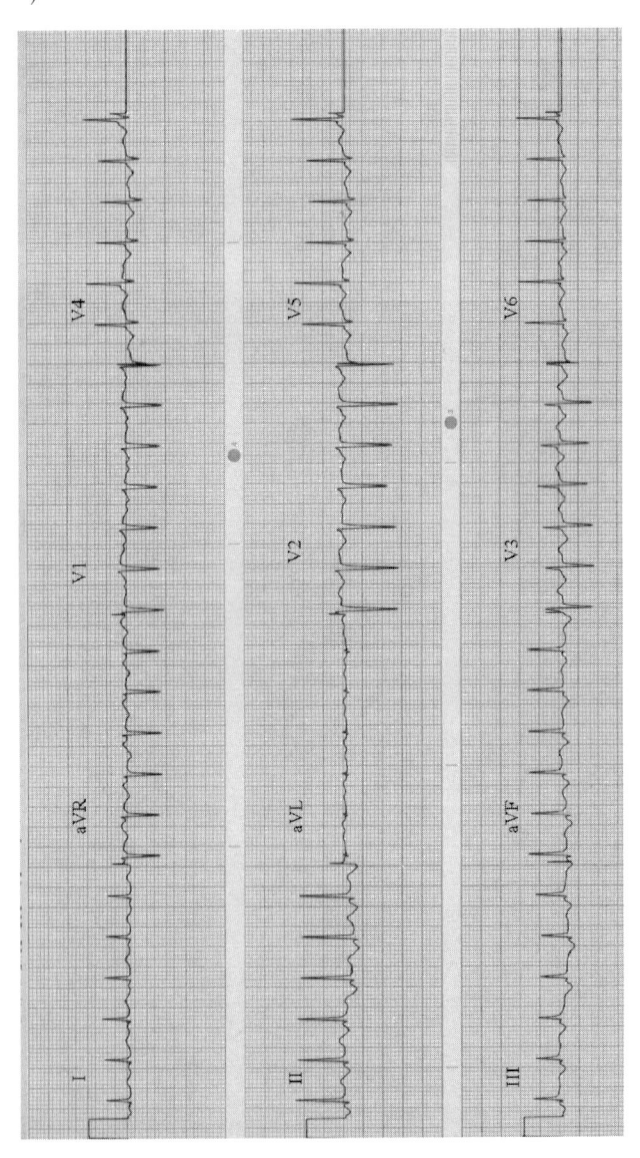

Fig. 1.2

1.10

Below is the ECG of an 81-year-old woman who is complaining of nausea and vomiting. On direct questioning she admits to taking 'heart pills'.

a) What are the tablets to which she is referring?
b) What complication has arisen?

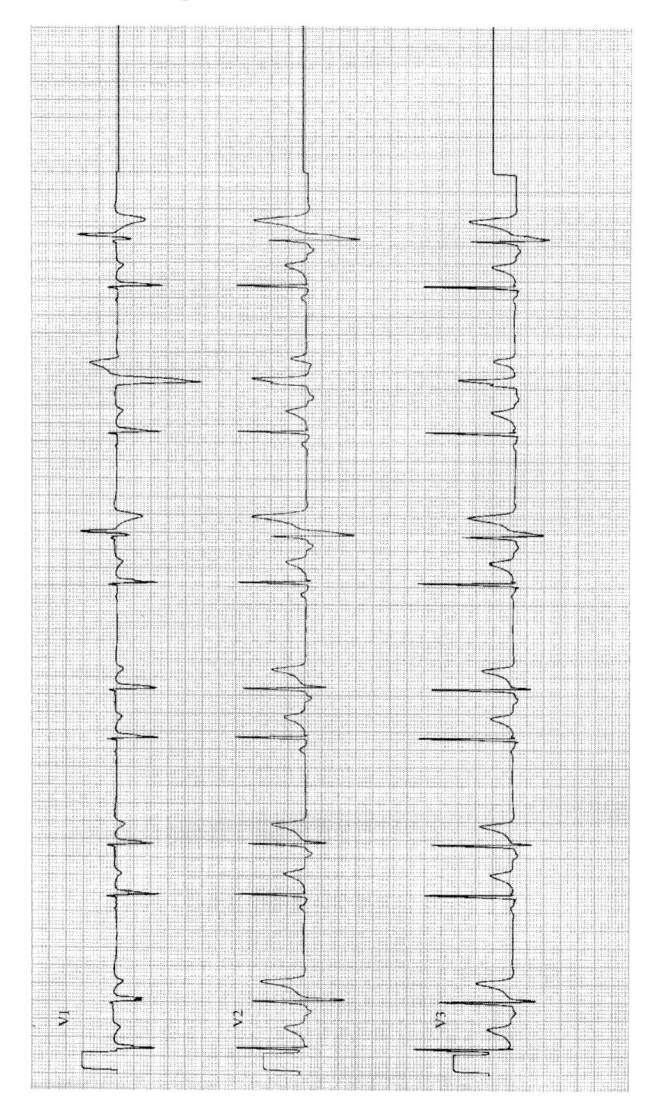

A → 112

Fig. 1.3

1.11

Below is the ECG of a 35-year-old man who is being investigated for bronchiectasis.

a) What is the ECG suggestive of?
b) What is the likely diagnosis?
c) What will an abdominal CT scan show?

A → 113

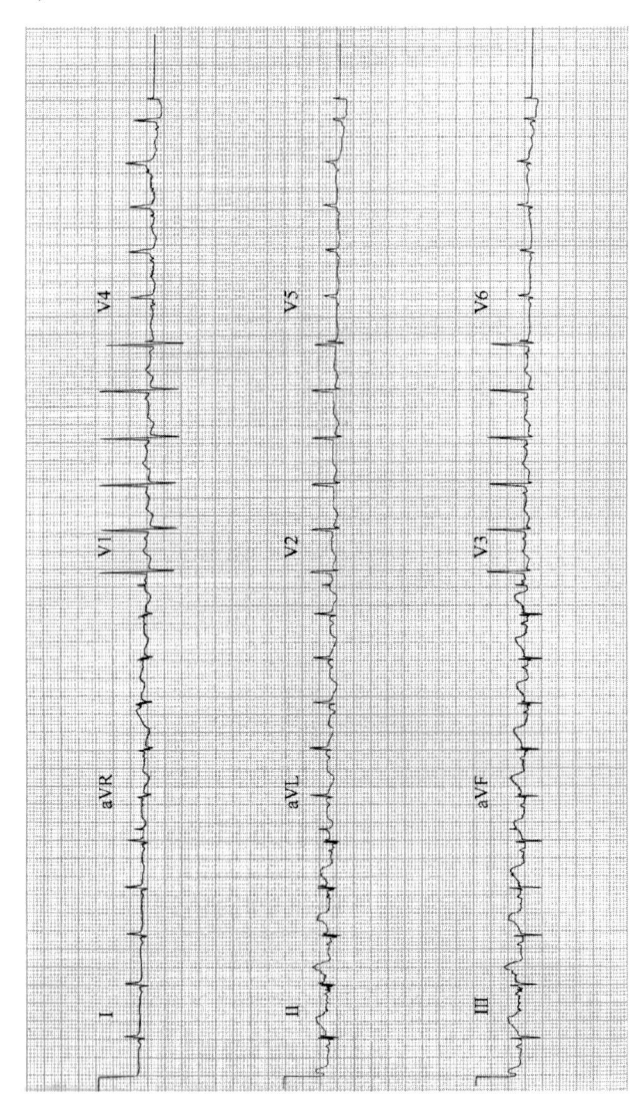

Fig. 1.4

CARDIOLOGY

1.12

A 25-year-old woman is being investigated for progressively worsening shortness of breath. Her ECG is shown below.

a) Name two abnormalities on the ECG.
b) What is the diagnosis?
c) List three possible causes.

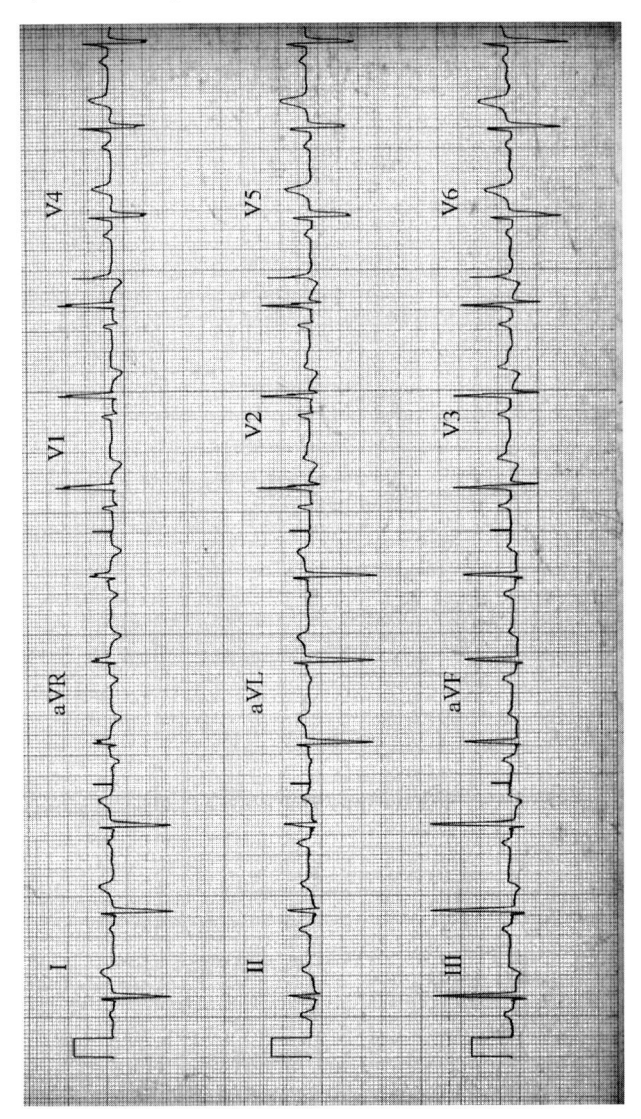

A → 113

Fig. 1.5

1.13

Below is the ECG of a 56-year-old man who has been brought to the Accident and Emergency department following a blackout.

a) What is the diagnosis?
b) What complication has occurred?

A → 115

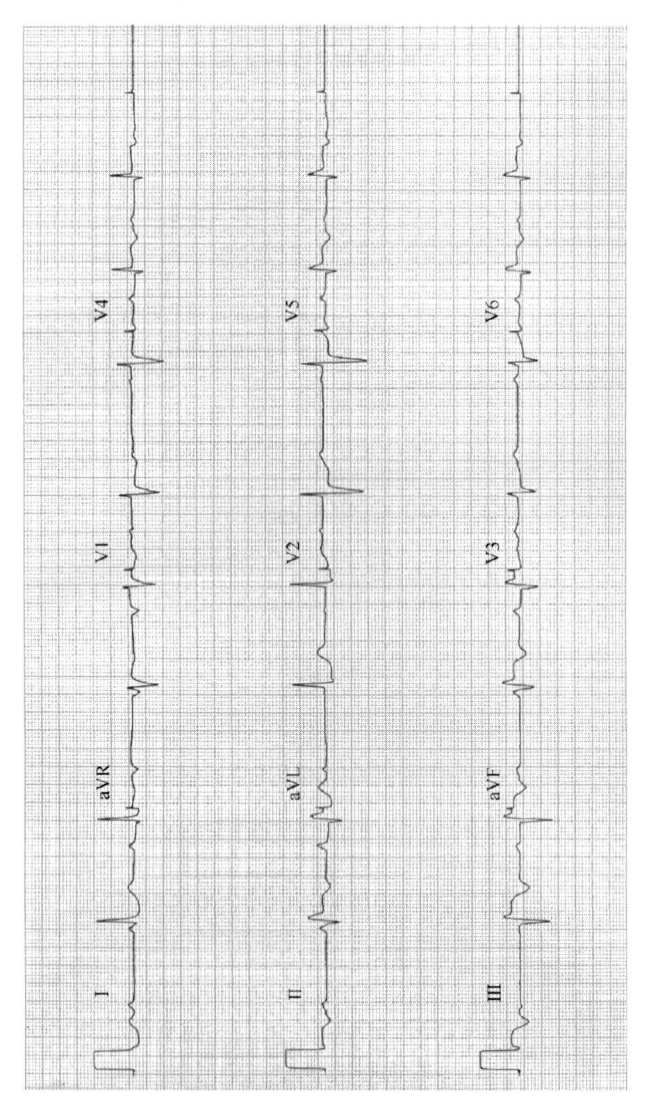

Fig. 1.6

1.14

Below is the ECG from an 84-year-old patient with acute on chronic renal failure. Shortly after this ECG was taken the patient had an asystolic cardiac arrest.

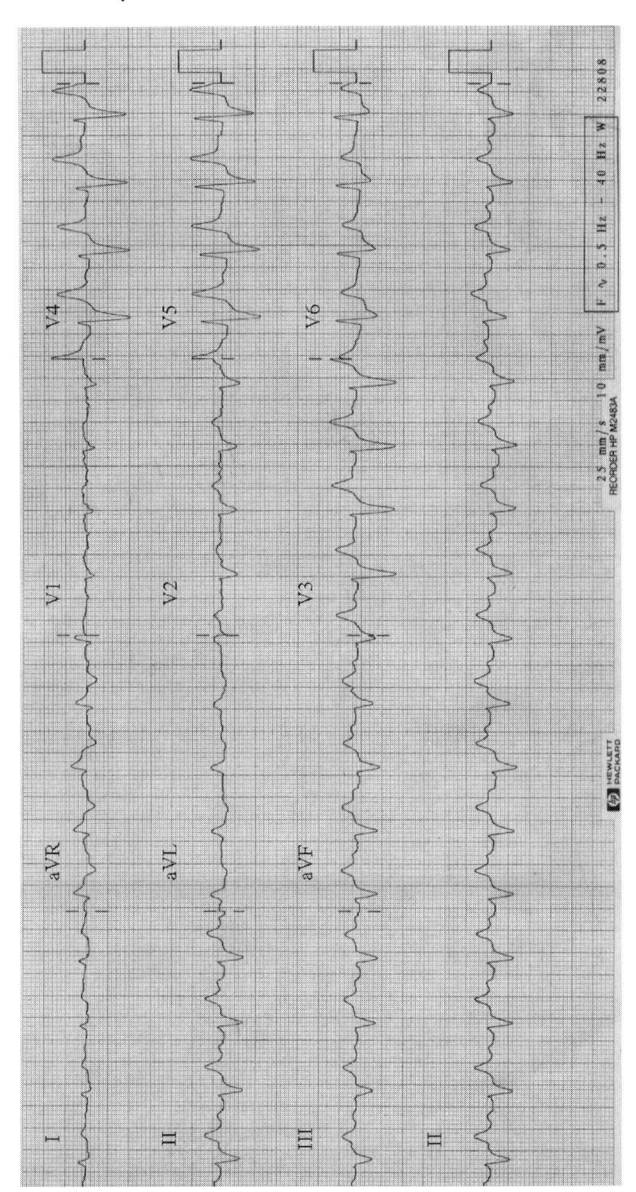

Fig. 1.7

a) Name two abnormalities present on the ECG.
b) What is the likely cause of the cardiac arrest?

1.15

The ECG below was taken from a 54-year-old man who collapsed suddenly in the street.

a) What is the cause of the collapse?

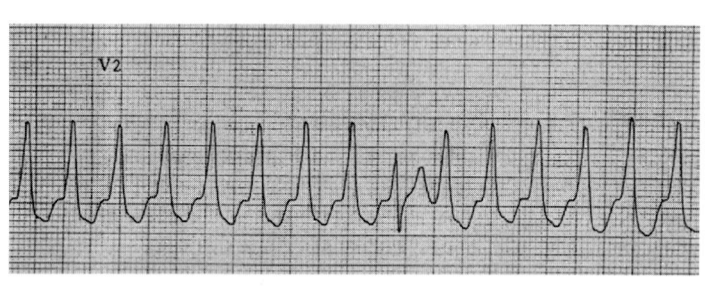

Fig. 1.8

1.16

Opposite is the ECG of a 65-year-old woman who presents with intermittent blackouts.

a) What does it show?
b) What treatment is indicated?

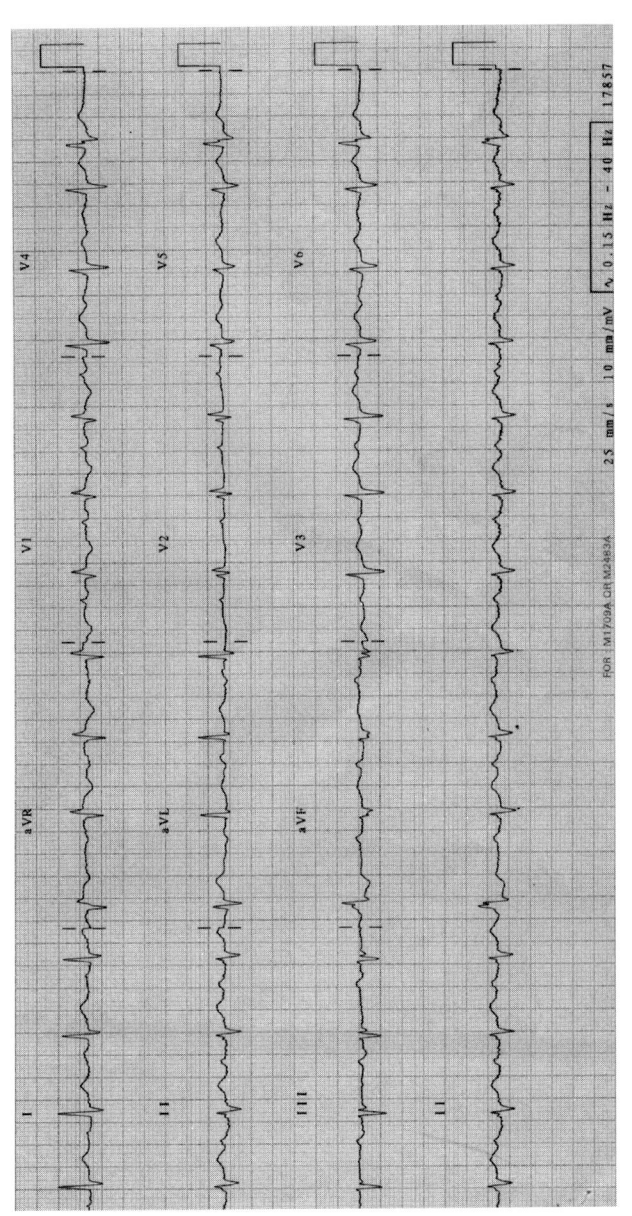

Fig. 1.9

1.17

Below is an ECG taken immediately after resuscitation of a 56-year-old man who has suffered a cardiac arrest. In the past he has suffered an inferolateral myocardial infarction and he is currently receiving treatment for paroxysmal atrial fibrillation.

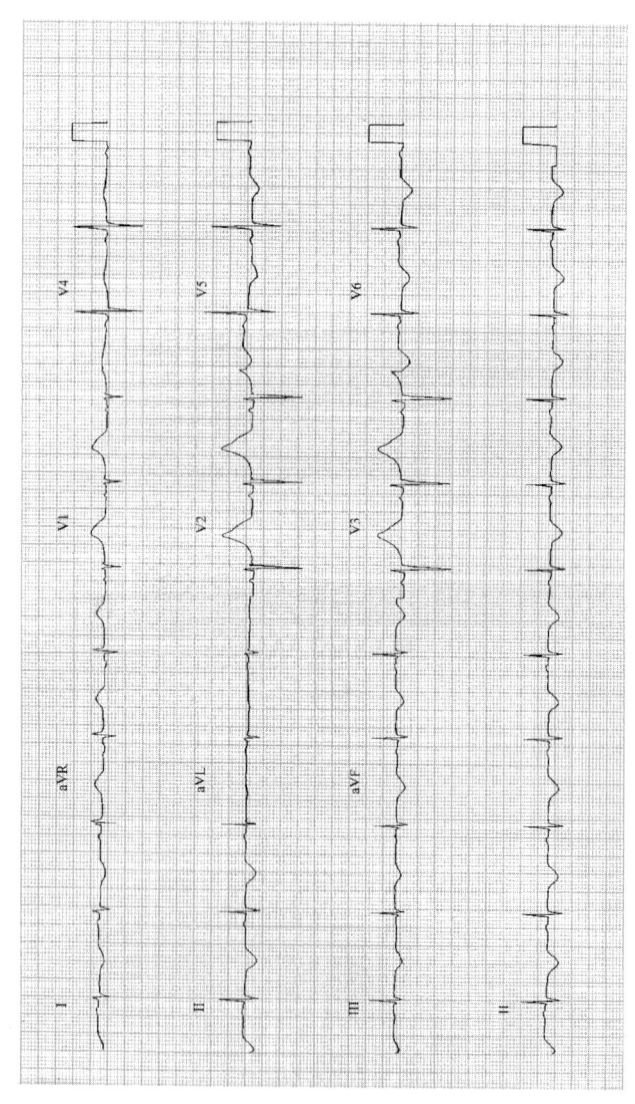

Fig. 1.10

a) In addition to the old MI what other abnormality does the ECG show?
b) What rhythm disturbance is suggested by the clinical data as a cause for the arrest?
c) What is the likely cause of this rhythm disturbance?

A → 117

1.18

A 25-year-old army recruit collapsed during circuit training. Medical assistance was close by and immediate ECG showed ventricular fibrillation from which he was successfully defibrillated. Below is the M-mode recording from a subsequent transthoracic echocardiogram.

a) Name two abnormalities.
b) What is the diagnosis?

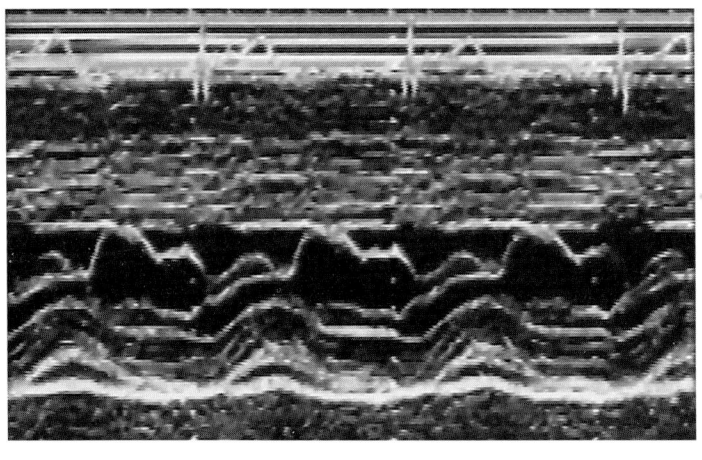

A → 122

Fig. 1.11

1.19

This is the M-mode echocardiogram of a 54-year-old man who presents with a left-sided hemiplegia.

a) What abnormalities are present on the echocardiogram?
b) What is the diagnosis?
c) What is the likely aetiology of the patient's symptoms?

A → 124

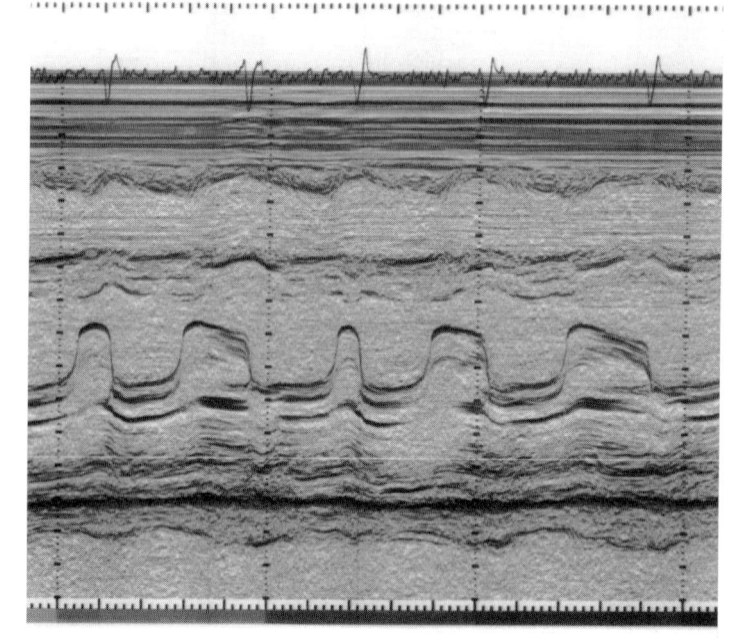

Fig. 1.12

1.20

Below are shown the M-mode recording and apical four-chamber view taken from the echocardiogram of a 45-year-old man who presents with worsening peripheral oedema. He is known to have small cell carcinoma of the bronchus and on examination is noted to have an abnormality of his JVP.

a) What diagnosis does the echocardiogram suggest?
b) What is the likely cause in this patient?
c) What is the abnormality of the JVP?

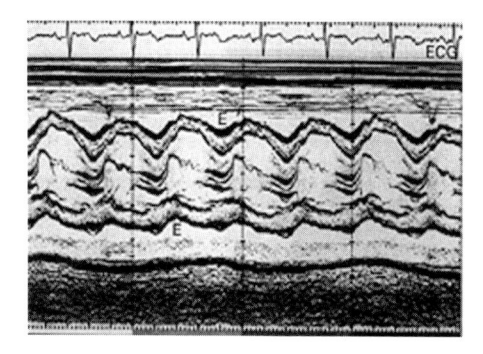

A → 125

Fig. 1.13 Reproduced by permission of A. J. Camm (P. J. Kumar and M. L. Clark, eds. 'Clinical Medicine', Baillière Tindall 1990)

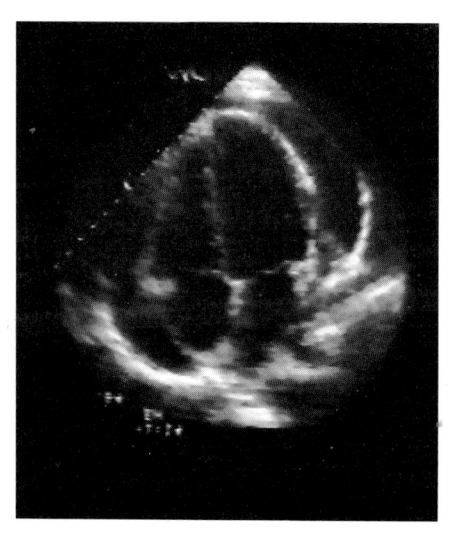

Fig. 1.14

1.21

A 55-year-old woman is referred to the cardiology department complaining of a three-month history of malaise, intermittent fever and weight loss. On examination she is found to have an added sound in early diastole with a mid-diastolic murmur. Below are the results from routine haematological tests and images from M-mode and 2D echocardiography in the parasternal long axis plane.

Hb	11.7 g/dL
WCC	6.4×10^9/L
Platelets	240×10^9/L
ESR	75 mm in 1 h

a) What is the diagnosis?
b) What investigation would you perform?

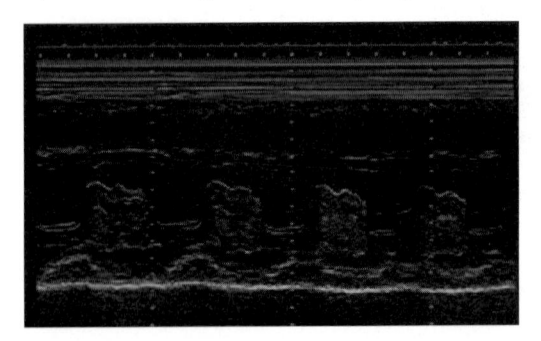

A → 127

Fig. 1.15

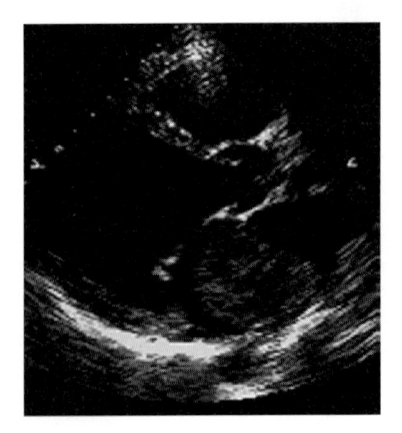

Fig. 1.16

CARDIOLOGY

1.22

Below is the 2D echocardiogram (apical four-chamber view) of a 63-year-old man who suffered an acute myocardial infarction 17 days ago.

a) What complication has developed?
b) What treatment is indicated?

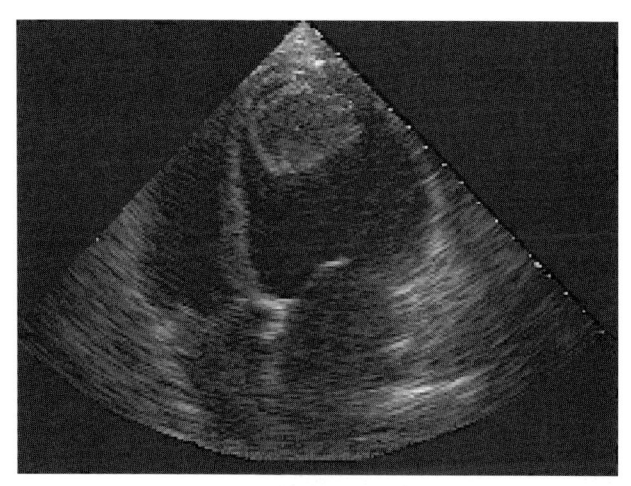

A → 130

Fig. 1.17

1.23

A 44-year-old man presents to the Accident and Emergency department two days after a prolonged episode of retrosternal chest pain. He now feels fine and has just 'popped in for a check-up'. He has no prior cardiac history and a physical examination is unremarkable. Below are his thallium scan and ECG.

A → 133

a) What is the diagnosis?
b) What immediate treatment would you give?

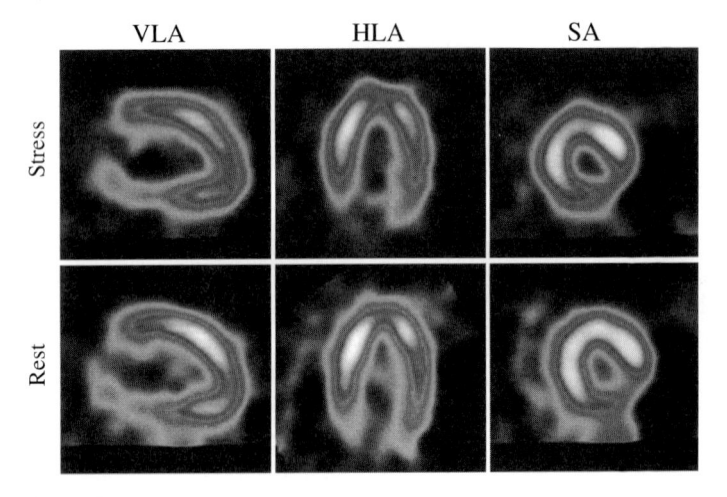

Fig. 1.18

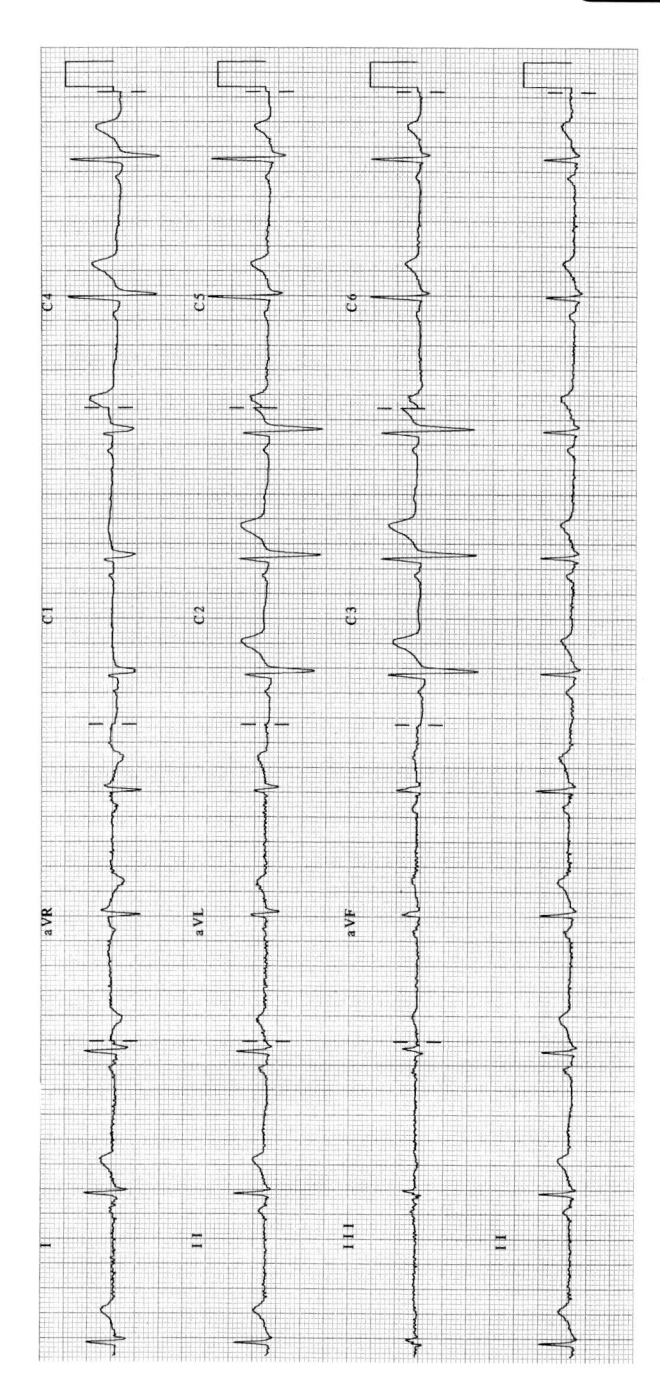

Fig. 1.19

2 ENDOCRINOLOGY

ENDOCRINOLOGY

2.1

A 55-year-old publican presents with weakness in his legs and shortness of breath.

Na	143 mmol/L
K	2.5 mmol/L
Urea	8.0 mmol/L
Glucose	9.6 mmol/L
Bicarbonate	35 mmol/L

a) What is a likely unifying diagnosis?
b) What cause is suggested by the data?
c) What three further investigations would you request?
d) Name five reasons why this patient may have leg weakness.

A → 136

2.2

A 35-year-old single mother of three young children is being investigated for weight gain and menstrual irregularity. She admits to drinking one bottle of gin per week and is finding it difficult to cope. A dexamethasone suppression test is performed.

	Time (min)	Plasma cortisol (nmol/L)
Overnight test: (2 mg dexamethasone at 22.00 h)	09.00 next day	600
High-dose test: (8 mg dexamethasone daily for two days)	09.00 day 1 09.00 day 2 09.00 day 3	980 450 250

a) Name two possible diagnoses.
b) What investigation would you do to distinguish between the two possible diagnoses?

A → 141

2.3

A 45-year-old man is referred with headache and blurred vision. He has recently been diagnosed as having chronic bronchitis. The results of routine blood tests and a high-dose dexamethasone suppression test are shown below.

	High-dose dexamethasone suppression test	
	Time (min)	Plasma cortisol (nmol/L)
(8 mg dexamethasone daily for two days)	09.00 day 1	890
	09.00 day 2	970
	09.00 day 3	920

a) Name two possible diagnoses.
b) What blood test would differentiate between these causes?

2.4

A 22-year-old woman presents with marked hirsutism, temporal balding, weight gain and amenorrhoea. Her BP is 170/110 and chest X-ray is normal.

Hb	16.2 g/dL	
WCC	7.6×10^9/L	
Platelets	223×10^9/L	
ESR	55 mm/h	
Na	138 mmol/L	
K	2.9 mmol/L	
Urea	6.2 mmol/L	
Midnight cortisol	900 nmol/L	
24h urine 17-ketosteroids	38 μmol/L	(normal 0–9)

	High-dose dexamethasone suppression test	
	Time (min)	Plasma cortisol (nmol/L)
(2 mg dexamethasone 6-hourly for two days)	09.00 day 1	980
	09.00 day 2	900
	09.00 day 3	750

a) What diagnosis does the data suggest?

ENDOCRINOLOGY

2.5

A 26-year-old woman is brought into casualty semiconscious. There has been a three-month history of weight loss, abdominal pain and general fatigue. The results of her blood and urine tests are shown below.

Na	128 mmol/L
K	6.8 mmol/L
Urea	14.0 mmol/L
Bicarbonate	12.8 mmol/L
Urine dipstick	Negative for blood, protein and glucose

a) What is the most likely diagnosis?
b) Name five possible causes.
c) What immediate treatment would you give?
d) What three further investigations would you perform?
e) What cardinal physical sign would you look for?

A → 142

2.6

A 45-year-old man presents with malaise, weight loss, nausea and dizziness on standing. He has a past history of ulcerative colitis but has been in remission for the past three months.

	Time	Plasma cortisol (nmol/L)
Short Synacthen test (Synacthen 0.25 mg)	0	88
	30 min	230
Long Synacthen test (1 mg daily for three days)	Day 1	250
	Day 2	370
	Day 3	800

a) What is the diagnosis?
b) Name two possible causes.
c) What further investigation would you do to distinguish between these causes?

A → 145

27

2.7

A 28-year-old woman presents with a six-month history of weight loss and diarrhoea. On examination she has a few discretely enlarged cervical and inguinal lymph nodes, and a tachycardia of 120 bpm. Investigations are as follows.

Hb	10.1 g/dL	
WCC	8.1 × 10⁹/L	
Platelets	152 × 10⁹/L	
MCV	101 fL	
Free T4	18.4 pmol/L	(normal 9.0–22.0)
TSH	< 0.2 mU/L	(normal 0.5–5.7)

A → 146

a) What further test would you perform?
b) What is the most likely diagnosis?

2.8

A 70-year-old man with longstanding rheumatoid arthritis is admitted with a five-day history of non-specific pain in the left side of his chest and a productive cough. He has a low-grade pyrexia (37.3°C) and is tachycardic (120 bpm). His chest X-ray shows consolidation at the left base.

Free T4	7.9 pmol/L	(normal 9.0–22.0)
Free T3	2.2 pmol/L	(normal 2.9–8.9)
TSH	0.2 mU/L	(normal 0.5–5.7)

A → 149

a) What is the most likely cause of this abnormality?
b) How would you investigate further?

2.9

A 25-year-old secretary presents with a four-month history of amenorrhoea and, more recently, vomiting. She admits to feeling hotter over the past few weeks and on examination she has a fine tremor. Her pulse is 125 bpm.

Total T4	190 nmol/L	(normal 70–140)
TSH	2.4 mU/L	(normal 0.5–5.7)

A → 151

a) What investigation would you request to confirm the diagnosis?

2.10

An 18-year-old girl is being treated with thyroxine for hypothyroidism. Six months after initiation of treatment her TFTs are as follows.

| Free T4 | 36 pmol/L | (normal 9.0–22.0) |
| TSH | 9.8 mU/L | (normal 0.5–5.7) |

a) What is the likely cause of these TFTs?

2.11

A 22-year-old woman presents with a painful swelling in the anterior aspect of her neck. She has noticed some palpitations and on examination she has a fine tremor.

Free T4	35 pmol/L	(normal 9.0–22.0)
TSH	< 0.2 mU/L	(normal 0.5–5.7)
ESR	110 mm/h	

a) What is the diagnosis?
b) What treatment is required?
c) What investigation will confirm the diagnosis?

2.12

A 35-year-old woman is referred to the endocrinologist for investigation of palpitations, weight loss and amenorrhoea. Her thyroid function is as follows.

Free T4	33.8 pmol/L	(normal 9.0–22.0)
Free T3	12.1 pmol/L	(normal 2.9–8.9)
TSH	7.1 mU/L	(normal 0.5–5.7)

a) Give two possible diagnoses.
b) Name two investigations to differentiate between them.

2.13

A 28-year-old woman is referred to the endocrine clinic complaining of excess facial hair, which has been present since her late teens but seems to have become worse over the past year or so. On questioning she admits to not having had a period for eight months. On examination her weight is 100 kg but no physical abnormalities are detected.

Serum testosterone	4.8 nmol/L	(normal 0.8–3.0)
Plasma 17(OH)-progesterone	3.2 nmol/L	(normal < 15)
FSH	5 U/L	(normal < 8)
LH	21 U/L	(normal < 6)
Urinary oxogenic steroids	46 μmol/24 h	(normal 21–66)

a) What is the most likely diagnosis?
b) What further investigation would you perform?
c) How would you treat her?

A → 153

2.14

A 19-year-old woman is referred for investigation of amenorrhoea. It has been twelve months since her last period. She has no past medical history and is not on any medication.

βHCG	2.0 U/L	(normal < 5)
FSH	66 U/L	(normal 1–10)
LH	45 U/L	(normal 2.5–21)
Oestradiol	90 pmol/L	(normal 500–1100 mid-cycle)

a) What is the most likely diagnosis?
b) What two further investigations would you perform?

A → 155

2.15

A 30-year-old man presents with erectile impotence and loss of libido. Recently he has noticed a clear discharge from his right nipple. Examination is normal and he is not taking any medication.

Testosterone	3.5 nmol/L	(normal 10–35)
FSH	1.1 U/L	(normal 1–7)
LH	1.0 U/L	(normal 1–10)
TSH	3.5 mU/L	(normal 0.5–5.5)

a) What further investigation would you perform?
b) What is the likely diagnosis?

A → 156

ENDOCRINOLOGY

2.16

A six-year-old boy is being investigated for generalized weakness and failure to thrive. His parents have noticed that he frequently wants to go to the toilet to pass water. Examination, including blood pressure, is normal.

Na	136 mmol/L	
K	3.0 mmol/L	
Urea	4.0 mmol/L	
Glucose	4.6 mmol/L	
Bicarbonate	33 mmol/L	
Ca (total)	2.31 mmol/L	
Phosphate	0.82 mmol/L	
Albumin	37 g/L	
24 h urine Na	90 mmol/24 h	(normal 100–250)
24 h urine K	250 mmol/24 h	(normal 14–120)
Mid-stream urine	Dipstick	normal
	Microscopy	normal
	Culture	no growth
Glucose tolerance test	Normal	

a) What is the likely diagnosis?
b) How would you confirm this?
c) Suggest two possible treatments.

A → 158

2.17

A 45-year-old man is referred for investigation of polyuria, polydipsia and nocturia. On repeated examinations his blood pressure has been found to be elevated. Examination is otherwise normal. Liver function tests are normal but the results of other investigations are shown below.

Na	150 mmol/L
K	3.0 mmol/L
Urea	7.2 mmol/L
Bicarbonate	34 mmol/L

Oral glucose tolerance test (75 g of glucose)

Time (hours)	Blood glucose (mmol/L)
0	5.6
0.5	9.7
1.0	14.0
1.5	8.6
2.0	7.3

a) What is the likely diagnosis?
b) How would you confirm it?
c) Name the two commonest causes of this diagnosis.
d) Name two investigations to distinguish between these causes.

A → 159

2.18

A six-year-old boy is referred to the paediatric department because his GP is concerned that he might be entering puberty prematurely. On examination he has a few tufts of pubic and axillary hair. His testes feel normal and are approximately 3 ml in volume on each side.

Na	128 mmol/L
K	5.7 mmol/L
Urea	7.2 mmol/L
Testosterone	8 nmol/L (normal < 0.35)

a) What is the likely diagnosis?
b) Name a differential diagnosis.
c) What three further investigations would you perform?

A → 161

2.19

A 24-year-old man is admitted following a grand-mal seizure in a supermarket. Below are the results of initial investigations.

Na	138 mmol/L
K	3.6 mmol/L
Urea	7.8 mmol/L
Creatinine	101 μmol/L
Calcium	1.40 mmol/L
Phosphate	1.78 mmol/L
Albumin	38 g/L
pO_2	12 kPa

a) What important test is missing from the above initial post-seizure biochemical screen?
b) Name three possible diagnoses.
c) What three investigations would you perform to differentiate between these diagnoses?
d) What ECG abnormality would you expect to see?

A → 164

2.20

A 46-year-old man is brought to the Accident and Emergency room complaining of severe central abdominal pain radiating through to his back and associated with pronounced retching and vomiting. He has been constipated for the past few months. Examination is normal apart from some bruising around the umbilicus.

Na	144 mmol/L	
K	5.8 mmol/L	
Urea	14 mmol/L	
Bicarbonate	18 mmol/L	
Calcium	3.60 mmol/L	
Phosphate	0.55 mmol/L	
Albumin	28 g/L	
Bilirubin (total)	7 μmol/L	(normal < 17)
AST	33 IU/L	(normal 13–42)
ALP	110 IU/L	(normal 40–115)
Gamma GT	80 IU/L	(normal < 40)

a) What additional acute investigation would you perform?
b) What is the likely cause of the acute presentation?
c) What is the likely unifying diagnosis and the most likely differential diagnosis?
d) What two investigations would you perform to differentiate between these diagnoses?

A → 165

2.21

A four-year-old girl is referred with failure to thrive. On examination she is below the 95th centile for height and has marked genu-valgum deformities.

Calcium	2.25 mmol/L	(normal for age 2.1–2.6)
Phosphate	0.75 mmol/L	(normal for age 1.29–1.78)
Albumin	38 g/L	
ALP	650 IU/L	(normal for age < 400)
Wrist X-ray	Cupped metaphyses with indistinct epiphyseal margins and widening of the epiphyses	

a) What is the diagnosis?
b) What investigation would you perform to support this diagnosis?
c) What is the treatment?

A → 167

ENDOCRINOLOGY

2.22

These are the results of a 24-year-old care assistant who is being investigated for recurrent dizzy spells and blackouts.

Na	138 mmol/L	
K	3.2 mmol/L	
Urea	5.2 mmol/L	
Glucose	2.1 mmol/L	
Bilirubin (total)	9 μmol/L	(normal < 17)
AST	17 IU/L	(normal 13–42)
ALP	101 IU/L	(normal 40–115)
Albumin	38 g/L	

a) Name two possible diagnoses.
b) What investigation would you perform to differentiate between them?

A → 168

2.23

A 55-year-old man presents with worsening peripheral oedema of three months' duration. He has had a number of referrals to respiratory physicians over the past three years for recurrent episodes of troublesome wheeze but pulmonary function tests and bronchoscopy were normal. In addition, his GP has diagnosed him as suffering from 'colitis' and he takes loperamide for the control of diarrhoea. On examination he appears flushed and has prominent CV waves in the JVP. Below are the results from cardiac catheterization.

	Pressure (mm Hg)	Saturation (%)
SVC	–	77
RA (mean)	12	80
RV	17/8	79
PA	17/8	81
LA (mean)	8	98
LV	115/0	96
Aorta	110/70	97

a) What investigation would you perform?
b) What is the unifying diagnosis?

A → 170

35

2.24

A 50-year-old man is being investigated for constant headaches and resistant hypertension. He has a past history of renal stones and multiple duodenal ulcers. He currently takes omeprazole 40 mg to relieve his symptoms of indigestion.

Na	135 mmol/L
K	4.0 mmol/L
Urea	9.1 mmol/L
Bicarbonate	28 mmol/L
Ca (total)	2.73 mmol/L
Phosphate	0.69 mmol/L
Albumin	37 g/L

Oral glucose tolerance test (75 g glucose)

Time (min)	Plasma glucose (mmol/L)	Growth hormone (mU/L)
0	5.2	8.2
30	9.6	15.6
60	12.5	25.5
90	9.8	16.4
120	8.1	7.8

a) What three endocrine abnormalities are evident from the data?
b) What other organ would you like to investigate in more detail?
c) What is a likely unifying diagnosis?

A → 170

2.25

A 35-year-old man is brought into the Accident and Emergency department with sudden onset of severe headache and palpitations. He has had two similar episodes in the past year but they have not been so severe. He has no relevant past medical history and is not on medication but several members of his family have had thyroidectomy. On examination he is sweaty with a sinus tachycardia of 130 bpm and a blood pressure of 180/100. There is a firm mass palpable in the lower pole of the left lobe of the thyroid. Examination is otherwise unremarkable.

ENDOCRINOLOGY

Na	137 mmol/L
K	3.2 mmol/L
Urea	6.8 mmol/L
Bicarbonate	29 mmol/L
Glucose	12.0 mmol/L
Ca (total)	2.8 mmol/L
Phosphate	0.60 mmol/L
Albumin	38 g/L
Hb	18.5 g/dL

a) What is the cause of the hypercalcaemia?
b) Name a likely unifying diagnosis.
c) What two investigations would you perform to confirm the diagnosis?
d) What immediate treatment would you give?

A → 172

2.26

A 55-year-old man is brought into hospital unconscious. His BP is 90/50 and his pulse is 50 bpm. Rectal temperature is 33.5°C and his ankle reflexes are a little slow to relax but examination is otherwise unremarkable. His wife says that he has looked quite pale for the past three months and he has not felt like having intercourse for the past six months, which is very unusual for him.

Hb	10.9 g/dL	
WCC	7.1×10^9/L	
Platelets	221×10^9/L	
MCV	103 fL	
Na	128 mmol/L	
K	5.3 mmol/L	
Urea	9.4 mmol/L	
Glucose	3.2 mmol/L	
Albumin	38 g/L	
Bilirubin	10 μmol/L	(normal < 17)
AST	65 IU/L	(normal 13–42)
LDH	327 IU/L	(normal 100–300)

a) What immediate investigations would you do (name six)?
b) What is the most likely diagnosis?
c) Give five aspects of your immediate management of this patient.

A → 173

37

3 HAEMATOLOGY

HAEMATOLOGY

3.1

A 28-year-old man was noted, by his wife, to be jaundiced three weeks after a flu-like illness. Subsequent investigation reveals the following results.

Hb	7.0 g/dL	
WCC	6.0×10^9/L	
Platelets	470×10^9/L	
Reticulocytes	7%	
Albumin	38 g/L	
Total bilirubin	38 µmol/L	(normal < 17)
AST	28 IU/L	(normal 13–42)
ALP	61 IU/L	(normal 40–115)
Urine dipstick	Urobilinogen: ++ positive	
	Bilirubin: negative	
	Noted to be dark	

a) What is the likely diagnosis?
b) Why is the urine dark?

A → 176

3.2

A 58-year-old man presents to the Accident and Emergency department with sudden onset of pleuritic chest pain and shortness of breath.

Hb	13.5 g/dL	
WCC	14.7 × 10⁹/L	
Neutrophils	71%	(normal 40–75%)
Lymphocytes	20%	(normal 20–45%)
Monocytes	2%	(normal 2–10%)
Basophils	6%	(normal 0–1%)
Eosinophils	1%	(normal 1–6%)
Platelets	550 × 10⁹/L	
RCC	5.6 × 10¹²/L	(normal 4.5–6.5)
MCH	21.1 pg	(normal 27–32)
MCHC	29 g/dL	(normal 31–35)
PCV	0.57	(normal 0.40–0.54)
MCV	69 fL	
Albumin	38 g/L	
Total bilirubin	38 µmol/L	(normal < 17)
AST	28 IU/L	(normal 13–42)
ALP	61 IU/L	(normal 40–115)
Urine dipstick	Urobilinogen: ++ positive Bilirubin: negative Noted to be dark	

a) Name two haematological abnormalities.
b) What is the probable unifying diagnosis?
c) What is the cause of the chest pain?
d) What four tests would you request to investigate the haematological abnormalities?
e) While in hospital the patient has two episodes of diplopia, each lasting for about 10 min. What is the cause of these episodes?

A → 177

HAEMATOLOGY

3.3

A 26-year-old woman presents to her GP with lethargy. Investigation reveals the following results.

Hb	11.6 g/dL	
WCC	4.8×10^9/L	
Platelets	232×10^9/L	
RCC	4.0×10^{12}/L	(normal 3.8–5.8)
PCV	0.57	(normal 0.37–0.47)
HbA$_2$	4.2%	(normal < 3.5%)

a) What is the likely diagnosis?
b) What two investigations would you request to confirm the diagnosis?
c) This patient is getting married shortly. What advice would you give her?

A → 178

3.4

An 18-year-old epileptic girl presents to her GP with lethargy of three months' duration.

Hb	9.8 g/dL	
WCC	6.2×10^9/L	
Platelets	110×10^9/L	
MCV	105 fL	
Albumin	38 g/L	
Bilirubin	17 µmol/L	(normal < 17)
AST	58 IU/L	(normal 13–42)
ALP	55 IU/L	(normal 40–115)
TSH	5.1 mU/L	(normal 0.5–5.5)

a) What further investigations would you do (name three)?
b) What is the likely diagnosis?
c) Why might her legs be weak?

A → 179

41

3.5

A 68-year-old woman is being investigated for recurrent chest infections.

Hb	8.4 g/dL
WCC	32.4 × 10⁹/L
Lymphocytes	26 × 10⁹/L
Platelets	192 × 10⁹/L
Blood film	Normochromic, normocytic with polychromasia

A → 180

a) What is the diagnosis?
b) What two complications may have occurred?
c) What three investigations would you perform?
d) What other characteristic feature might be seen on a blood film?

3.6

A 27-year-old woman is admitted via the Accident and Emergency department with a painful swollen left calf. The results of her coagulation screen are shown.

PT	13 s	(control = 13)
TT	13 s	(control = 12)
KPTT	92 s	(control = 35)

The KPTT does not correct after mixing with normal plasma.

A → 180

a) What is the likely cause of the clotting abnormality?

3.7

An 11-year-old boy is noted to bleed excessively during an appendicectomy operation. His clotting results are as follows.

PT	14 s	(control = 13)
TT	13 s	(control = 12)
KPTT	75 s	(control = 35)
Bleeding time	14 min	(normal 2–8 min)

A → 181

a) What is the most likely diagnosis?
b) How would you confirm it?

3.8

A two-year-old boy develops a haemarthrosis following a minor fall at home. His coagulation studies are as follows.

PT	12 s	(control = 13)
TT	13 s	(control = 12)
KPTT	89 s	(control = 35)
Factor VIIIc activity	normal	

a) What is the most likely diagnosis?
b) What investigation will confirm this?

A → 182

3.9

Following a TURP for prostatic cancer with bladder outflow obstruction, the patient continues to pass large amounts of blood and clots. The results of his investigations are as follows.

Hb	8.7 g/dL	
WCC	$17.2 \times 10^9/L$	
Platelets	$76 \times 10^9/L$	
INR	3.2	
KPTT	120 s	(control = 35)

a) What is the most likely cause of the clotting abnormality?
b) What further investigations would you perform (name three)?

A → 182

3.10

This is the bone marrow cytochemistry of a 45-year-old woman with pancytopenia.

Sudan black	+
Myeloperoxidase	+
Periodic acid schiff (PAS)	−
Non-specific esterase (NSE)	++

a) What is the diagnosis?

A → 183

3.11

A 14-year-old girl presents to her GP with a three-week history of malaise and sore throat. On examination she is found to have cervical lymphadenopathy. Her investigations are as follows.

Paul–Bunnell test	Agglutination with sheep red cells
No absorption	+
After absorption on guinea-pig kidney	+
After absorption on ox cells	–

| Anti EBV IgG | negative |
| Anti EBV IgM | negative |

(EBV = Epstein–Barr Virus)

a) Name three possible diagnoses.
b) What is the most important investigation to do next?
c) Name three further investigations.

3.12

A six-year-old child with sickle-cell disease develops worsening shortness of breath on exertion over a period of just a few days.

Hb	4.5 g/dL	
WCC	6.8×10^9/L	
Platelets	352×10^9/L	
MCH	28.0 pg	(normal 27–32)
MCHC	35 g/dL	(normal 31–35)
MCV	81 fL	
Reticulocytes	0.1%	

a) What is the most likely diagnosis?

3.13

A 58-year-old man presents to his GP with a general malaise of two weeks' duration and recent onset of prolonged nose bleeds. His past medical history consists only of Hodgkin's lymphoma, 10 years earlier, for which he was treated with chlorambucil.

Hb	8.3 g/dL	
WCC	68.3×10^9/L	
Platelets	23×10^9/L	
Blood film	Schistocytes present	
PT	18 s	(control = 13)
TT	23 s	(control = 12)
APTT	70 s	(control = 35)
Fibrinogen	60 mg/dL	(normal 150–400)

a) What is the probable diagnosis?
b) What complication has occurred?
c) What three further investigations would you perform?

A → 186

3.14

A six-year-old boy was brought to the Accident and Emergency department with prolonged epistaxis. Two weeks' earlier he had been treated by his GP with antibiotics for a sore throat.

Hb	11.1 g/dL	
WCC	9.0×10^9/L	
Platelets	18×10^9/L	
PT	14 s	(control = 13)
TT	11 s	(control = 12)
APTT	38 s	(control = 35)
Blood film	Normal apart from thrombocytopenia	

a) What is the most likely diagnosis?
b) What two further investigations would you perform?

A → 186

3.15

A 30-year-old woman who is 28 weeks' pregnant suddenly collapses and on arrival at hospital is found to have a mild left-sided hemiplegia and diffuse purpura on her legs. Investigations are as follows.

Hb	8.4 g/dL	
WCC	10.0×10^9/L	
Platelets	28×10^9/L	
PT	14 s	(control = 13)
TT	12 s	(control = 12)
APTT	33 s	(control = 35)
Na	142 mmol/L	
K	5.6 mmol/L	
Urea	27.8 mmol/L	
Creatinine	210 µmol/L	
Blood film	Fragmented red cells and some spherocytes	
Direct Coombs' test	Negative	

a) What is the diagnosis?

3.16

A 24-year-old man, who is being treated for dermatitis herpetiformis, is noticed by his girlfriend to be jaundiced. Subsequent investigations are shown below.

Hb	9.2 g/dL	
WCC	11.0×10^9/L	
Platelets	430×10^9/L	
MCV	108 fL	
Reticulocytes	4.2%	
Albumin	38 g/L	
Bilirubin	33 µmol/L	(normal < 17)
AST	25 IU/L	(normal 13–42)
ALP	60 IU/L	(normal 40–115)
Blood film	Fragmented red cells and some macrocytes	

a) What is the likely diagnosis?
b) What else may be seen on the blood film?
c) Name two other factors that might be contributing to the anaemia.

HAEMATOLOGY

3.17

An 18-year-old girl is brought to casualty with severe nausea and vomiting. She has had diarrhoea for the past week, which she put down to an Indian takeaway meal. On examination she is found to be unwell, tachypnoeic and hypertensive with a blood pressure of 180/110.

Hb	8.2 g/dL	
WCC	7.8 × 10⁹/L	
Platelets	37 × 10⁹/L	
Na	138 mmol/L	
K	6.2 mmol/L	
Urea	26.2 mmol/L	
Creatinine	240 μmol/L	
Albumin	35 g/L	
Bilirubin	27 μmol/L	(normal < 17)
AST	30 IU/L	(normal 13–42)
ALP	62 IU/L	(normal 40–115)

a) Name two differential diagnoses.
b) Name three investigations to distinguish between them.
c) Name three further investigations.
d) What is a possible cause of her tachypnoea?

A → 189

47

3.18

A 12-year-old boy visits his GP's travel clinic for vaccinations and malaria prophylaxis. He is due to return to the Gambia to visit his grandparents. In the past he has had several episodes of jaundice but following normal liver enzymes and a normal liver ultrasound scan his parents have been reassured that he is probably just suffering from Gilbert syndrome.

Hb	11.8 g/dL	
WCC	6.7×10^9/L	
Platelets	350×10^9/L	
MCH	29 pg	(normal 27–32)
MCHC	37 g/dL	(normal 31–35)
MCV	89 fL	
Reticulocytes	3.9%	
Albumin	37 g/L	
Bilirubin	25 µmol/L	(normal < 17)
AST	35 IU/L	(normal 13–42)
ALP	70 IU/L	(normal 40–115)
Urine dipstick	Negative for bilirubin	

a) What is the probable diagnosis?
b) Name an alternative diagnosis.
c) What two investigations would you perform?
d) What would you advise the parents about travelling to Africa?

A → 189

3.19

A 58-year-old publican is being treated for pulmonary tuberculosis. Follow-up blood tests reveal the following.

Hb	9.1 g/dL
WCC	7.1×10^9/L
Platelets	171×10^9/L
MCV	106 fL
Blood film	Microspherocytes seen

a) What will be seen on bone marrow examination?

A → 191

HAEMATOLOGY

3.20

A 45-year-old businessman is on a business trip to Saudi Arabia. Shortly after arrival he develops a blistering rash on his face and fingers. He had a similar rash last summer.

Hb	12.1 g/dL	
WCC	7.8 × 10⁹/L	
Platelets	80 × 10⁹/L	
Albumin	30 g/L	
Bilirubin	15 µmol/L	(normal < 17)
AST	35 IU/L	(normal 13–42)
ALP	80 IU/L	(normal 40–115)
Gamma GT	85 IU/L	(normal < 40)
Ferritin	900 µg/L	(normal < 300)

a) What is the probable diagnosis?
b) What two investigations would you do?
c) What treatment may be of benefit?

A → 192

3.21

A 26-year-old woman is admitted to casualty following an epileptic seizure. She has had crampy abdominal pains for the past three days, and for the past week she has been taking cotrimoxazole for treatment of a urinary tract infection. This is her first seizure.

Hb	12.1 g/dL	
WCC	9.8 × 10⁹/L	
Platelets	370 × 10⁹/L	
Na	128 mmol/L	
K	4.1 mmol/L	
Urea	6.6 mmol/L	
Creatinine	100 µmol/L	
Albumin	37 g/L	
Bilirubin	22 µmol/L	(normal < 17)
AST	82 IU/L	(normal 13–42)
ALP	110 IU/L	(normal 40–115)

a) What is the diagnosis?
b) What three investigations would you perform?
c) What else is a priority?

A → 192

3.22

A six-year-old child is brought to the Accident and Emergency department with severe abdominal pain. He has no past medical history. On examination he is found to have a left-sided common peroneal nerve palsy.

Hb	9.8 g/dL
WCC	7.1×10^9/L
Platelets	331×10^9/L
Na	136 mmol/L
K	4.7 mmol/L
Urea	6.2 mmol/L
Blood film	Mild hypochromia and punctate basophilia
Urine	δALA positive PBG negative

a) What is the diagnosis?
b) Name one differential diagnosis.
c) What three investigations would you perform?

4 RENAL MEDICINE

4.1

A 50-year-old man presents with swollen ankles.

Na	128 mmol/L
K	3.7 mmol/L
Urea	6.8 mmol/L
Creatinine	110 μmol/L
Glucose	5.4 mmol/L
Albumin	22 g/L
Urinary protein	7.5 g/24 h
Renal biopsy Electron microscopy:	Thickening of basement membrane with subepithelial electron-dense deposits separated by spikes of basement membrane

a) What is the diagnosis?
b) Name two possible causes.
c) His renal function two weeks after presentation is shown below. What complication may have developed?

Na	129 mmol/L
K	6.5 mmol/L
Urea	30.0 mmol/L
Creatinine	550 μmol/L

A → 196

RENAL MEDICINE

4.2

Below are the results of urgent investigations that have been performed on a 67-year-old man who is two days post-transurethral resection of the prostate. The immediate post-operative period was complicated by acute haemorrhage during which the patient's blood pressure dropped to 60/40 mm HG for 45 min. He is catheterized and is draining small volumes of urine. The pre-operative urea and electrolytes were normal.

Plasma
Na	138 mmol/L
K	5.7 mmol/L
Urea	24.0 mmol/L
Creatinine	280 µmol/L

Urine
Sodium	15 mmol/L
Urea	240 mmol/L
Osmolarity	750 mosmol/L

a) What cause for this patient's acute renal failure is suggested by the above results?
b) What two investigations are indicated?

A → 197

4.3

A 12-year-old boy is taken to the GP by his mother because she is worried that his urine is red in colour. The child has been unwell for two days with a sore throat, fever, myalgia and loin pain.

Na	138 mmol/L
K	5.5 mmol/L
Urea	11.0 mmol/L
Creatinine	130 µmol/L
Urine dipstick	Blood +++
	Protein +++

a) What is the likely diagnosis?
b) What test would you perform to confirm this diagnosis?
c) What will this test show?

A → 198

4.4

A 45-year-old man is found to have haematuria and proteinuria on routine dipstick testing. On examination there is loss of subcutaneous fat affecting the face and arms.

Na	141 mmol/L
K	4.8 mmol/L
Urea	12.0 mmol/L
Creatinine	250 µmol/L
Serum C3	Reduced
Serum C4	Normal
Urine microscopy	Red cell casts; no organisms seen

a) What diagnosis does the above data suggest?
b) Name two differential diagnoses.
c) What three investigations would you perform to distinguish between the diagnoses?
d) What is the cause of the low C3?

4.5

A 30-year-old woman presents to the genitourinary clinic because she is concerned about the risks of having had unprotected intercourse with a casual acquaintance three weeks earlier.

High vaginal, endocervical urethral and rectal swabs	Negative	
VDRL	Positive	
TPHA	Negative	
Urine dipstick	+++ protein + glucose	
Urine culture	Negative	
ESR	50 mm/h	
CRP	4 mg/L	(normal < 10)
Hb	12.5 g/dL	
WBC	7.2×10^9/L	
Platelets	80×10^9/L	
Fasting glucose	5.5 mmol/L	

a) What is the likely diagnosis?
b) What three further tests would you perform?

4.6

A 45-year-old man is being investigated for hypertension. Below is the result of his isotope renogram ([$^{99}Tc^m$] DTPA).

a) What is the diagnosis?
b) What will an IVP show?
c) What additional investigation is required?

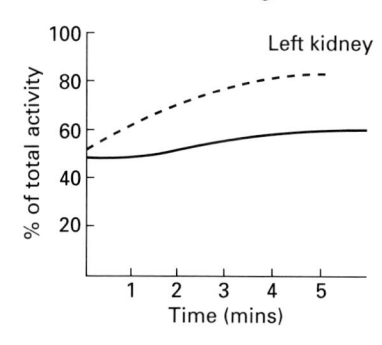

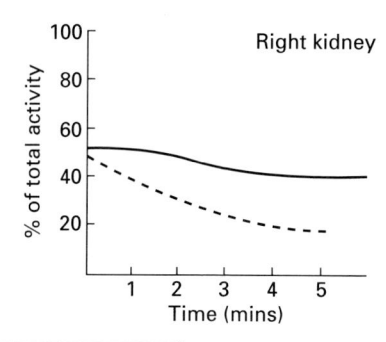

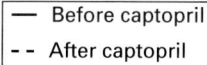

A → 202

Fig. 4.1

— Before captopril
-- After captopril

4.7

A 27-year-old woman presents with thirst, polyuria and polydipsia. She sustained a head injury six months ago and her symptoms began shortly after that. There is no other PMH of note and examination is normal.

Na	131 mmol/L
K	3.7 mmol/L
Urea	2.0 mmol/L
Glucose	5.4 mmol/L
Plasma osmolality	276.8 mOsm/kg
Urine osmolality	150 mOsm/kg
24h urine volume	8 litres

A → 203

a) What is the diagnosis?
b) How would you confirm it?

4.8

A 40-year-old male presents with a three-month history of thirst, polyuria and polydipsia. Chest X-ray shows honeycomb appearances of both lung fields together with a single lytic lesion in the shaft of the right humerus. The results of a water deprivation test are shown below.

Time (hours)	Plasma osmolality (mOsm/kg)	Urine osmolality (mOsm/kg)
0	288	110
3	297	120
6	310	120
8	310	135
DDAVP given		
10	320	350

A → 204

a) What is the cause of the results of the water deprivation test?
b) What is the unifying diagnosis?

RENAL MEDICINE

4.9

A 45-year-old female is referred by her GP with a six-month history of urinary frequency. She has had recurrent urinary tract infections in the past but these have always settled following antibiotics. She also has non-insulin-dependent diabetes for which she takes a sulphonylurea. The GP has prescribed two different courses of antibiotics for the current episode with no improvement in her symptoms. The results of the patient's water deprivation test are shown below.

Time (hours)	Plasma osmolality (mOsm/kg)	Urine osmolality (mOsm/kg)
0	292	118
3	305	122
6	310	115
8	310	130
DDAVP given		
10	308	128
Blood glucose	7.4 mmol/L	

a) What is the diagnosis?
b) Name two possible causes that are consistent with the patient's history.

A → 205

4.10

A 50-year-old businessman presents with an eight-week history of polyuria and polydipsia. He has no past medical history and is not on prescribed medication. He has, however, been under a lot of stress at work over the past few months and has required regular painkillers for frequent headaches. The results of his water deprivation test are shown below.

Time (hours)	Plasma osmolality (mOsm/kg)	Urine osmolality (mOsm/kg)
0	285	300
3	288	330
6	291	400
8	298	500
DDAVP given		
10	298	600

a) What is the diagnosis?

A → 205

4.11

A 28-year-old insulin-dependent diabetic is brought into casualty following a grand-mal seizure. His GP has been treating him with antibiotics for shortness of breath and a dry cough. He is teetotal.

Na	118 mmol/L
K	3.9 mmol/L
Urea	6.5 mmol/L
Creatinine	110 μmol/L
Glucose	9.5 mmol/L
Urine osmolality	580 mOsm/kg

a) What is the diagnosis?
b) What is the cause?

A → 206

4.12

A 54-year-old man is brought to casualty following a convulsion. He has no PMH and takes no medications. The results of his biochemistry tests are as follows.

Na	135 mmol/L
K	3.7 mmol/L
Urea	2.0 mmol/L
Glucose	5.5 mmol/L
Urine osmolality	570 mOsm/kg
Plasma osmolality	328 mOsm/kg

a) What is the likely cause of this man's seizure?

A → 207

RENAL MEDICINE

4.13

An 80-year-old man is found lying unconscious in his garden following a fall. He has been there all night. His temperature is 31°C and his blood pressure is 70/40 mm Hg. Biochemistry and arterial blood gas results are shown below.

Na	158 mmol/L
K	5.8 mmol/L
Urea	22.0 mmol/L
Chloride	105.0 mmol/L
Glucose	9.6 mmol/L
CK	150 IU/L
paO_2	10.2 kPa
$paCO_2$	2.9 kPa
Bicarbonate	12 mmol/L

a) What acid-base disturbance is present?
b) What is the probable cause?
c) What test would you do to confirm this?

A → 209

4.14

A 58-year-old heavy smoker with a long history of recurrent chest infections is admitted for an inguinal hernia repair. Blood gases performed as part of his pre-operative assessment were as follows.

paO_2	8.2 kPa
$paCO_2$	7.8 kPa
Bicarbonate	44 mmol/L
pH	7.38

a) What acid-base disturbance is present?

A → 210

4.15

A 34-year-old insulin-dependent diabetic is found semiconscious by a neighbour. He is a known alcoholic. On examination he is pyrexial at 38.5°C and has coarse crepitations at the base of his right lung.

Na	145 mmol/L
K	5.4 mmol/L
Urea	10.0 mmol/L
Glucose	25.0 mmol/L
paO_2	7.8 kPa
$paCO_2$	7.2 kPa
Bicarbonate	15 mmol/L
pH	7.12

A → 210

a) What acid-base disturbance is present?
b) What is the most likely cause?

4.16

These are the results of a 39-year-old man who is being investigated for recurrent renal stones.

Na	142 mmol/L
K	2.7 mmol/L
Urea	6.8 mmol/L
Creatinine	111 µmol/L
Calcium	2.05 mmol/L
Phosphate	0.70 mmol/L
Albumin	42 g/L

A → 210

a) What is the diagnosis?
b) Name two causes.
c) Will the chloride be normal, high or low?

4.17

A 42-year-old man with a long history of alcohol abuse is admitted unwell with recurrent vomiting. He has no known PMH and his only medication is aluminium hydroxide, which he takes for indigestion.

Na	128 mmol/L
K	–
Urea	30 mmol/L
Glucose	6.1 mmol/L
pH	7.53
$paCO_2$	6.8 kPa
Bicarbonate	50 mmol/L

a) What is the cause of the acid-base disturbance?
b) Will the K^+ be high, low or normal?

A → 211

4.18

A 22-year-old woman is admitted with a seven-day history of profuse diarrhoea. The results of her blood tests are as follows.

Na	138 mmol/L
K	3.2 mmol/L
Urea	12 mmol/L
Chloride	112 mmol/L
$paCO_2$	2.9 kPa
Bicarbonate	15 mmol/L
pH	7.38

a) What acid-base disturbance is present?
b) Name three other causes.

A → 212

4.19

These are the results of a two-year-old girl who is being investigated for delayed walking and failure to thrive.

Na	142 mmol/L
K	2.6 mmol/L
Urea	6.4 mmol/L
Chloride	114 mmol/L
Glucose	5.4 mmol/L
Bicarbonate	14 mmol/L
Urine dipstick	++ to glucose

a) What is the likely diagnosis?
b) Name three causes.
c) How would you confirm the diagnosis?
d) What other test would you perform?

A → 212

4.20

A four-year-old boy is found unconscious by his mother. He has vomited several times. He is apyrexial and there is no obvious sign of infection although he appears short of breath.

Hb	15.0 g/dL
WCC	6.0×10^9/L
Platelets	332×10^9/L
Na	129 mmol/L
K	5.2 mmol/L
Urea	9.0 mmol/L
Glucose	3.2 mmol/L
paO$_2$	11.5 kPa
paCO$_2$	3.2 kPa
Bicarbonate	12 mmol/L
pH	7.15
Urine clinitest	positive

a) What investigation would aid diagnosis?
b) What is the diagnosis?

A → 213

4.21

A 65-year-old man is admitted with shortness of breath. His only PMH is that he has glaucoma.

Na	141 mmol/L
K	3.1 mmol/L
Urea	9.0 mmol/L
Chloride	120 mmol/L
paCO$_2$	2.8 kPa
Bicarbonate	14 mmol/L
pH	7.15

a) What acid-base disturbance is present?
b) What is the likely cause?

5 RHEUMATOLOGY

RHEUMATOLOGY

5.1

Below are the results of a 45-year-old man who has been referred to the ophthalmology clinic for assessment of diplopia of recent onset. He has also been referred to the ENT consultant for investigation of recurrent sinusitis and otitis media. Initial routine bloods are as follows.

Hb	10.2 g/dL
WCC	16.2×10^9/L (80% neutrophils)
Platelets	570×10^9/L
ESR	80 mm/h
Na	138 mmol/L
K	3.7 mmol/L
Urea	17 mmol/L
Creatinine	180 μmol/L
Urine dipstick	++ positive for red blood cells ++ positive for protein

These results prompted the further investigations shown below.

Rheumatoid factor	Positive	
ANA	Negative	
IgA	7.2 g/L	(normal 0.8–4.0)
IgG	22.3 g/L	(normal 5.3–16.5)
IgM	4.2 g/L	(normal 0.5–2.0)
Urine microscopy	Red cells, white cells and red cell casts	

a) What is the likely diagnosis?
b) What further tests would you do to confirm the diagnosis (name two)?

A → 218

65

5.2

A 45-year-old woman is referred to the dermatologist for investigation of a purpuric rash affecting her legs. Routine blood tests reveal the following.

Hb	12.2 g/dL
WCC	13.4 × 10⁹/L
Platelets	600 × 10⁹/L
Na	140 mmol/L
K	3.9 mmol/L
Urea	9.0 mmol/L
Creatinine	130 µmol/L
LFTs abnormal	

Subsequent blood tests are as follows.

HBsAg	Negative	
HCV RNA (by PCR)	Positive	
HAV IgM	Negative	
IgA	0.4 g/L	(normal 0.8–4.0)
IgG	2.4 g/L	(normal 5.3–16.5)
IgM	0.2 g/L	(normal 0.5–2.0)
C3	Reduced	
C4	Reduced	

A → 219

a) What diagnosis is suggested by the data?
b) What three further tests would you do?

5.3

A 50-year-old man is referred to the outpatient clinic for investigation of abnormal renal and liver function tests. He gives a three-month history of malaise and weight loss with intermittent, colicky abdominal pain after meals. On examination he has a purpuric rash affecting his shins and a blood pressure of 180/100. The results of subsequent investigations are shown below.

HBsAG	Positive
Rheumatoid factor	Negative
ANA	Negative
ANCA	Negative
ESR	75 mm/h

a) What is the most likely diagnosis?
b) Name a differential diagnosis.

A → 220

c) What three further investigations would you perform?

RHEUMATOLOGY

5.4

A 65-year-old woman presents to her GP with a two-month history of malaise, fatigue, headache, and pain and stiffness affecting her neck and shoulders. She has also noticed pain in her jaw and tongue on chewing food, which disappears after swallowing. On examination she has a temperature of 38°C and is tender to palpation over her shoulders, upper arms and neck.

Hb	11.5 g/dL	
WBC	7.8×10^9/L	
Platelets	243×10^9/L	
ESR	110 mm/h	
CK	90 IU/L	(normal 25–175)
Blood culture (× 2)	Negative	
Urine culture	Negative	

a) What is the probable diagnosis?
b) What immediate treatment would you give?
c) What further investigation would you perform?
d) What is the likely cause of her anaemia?

A → 221

5.5

A 36-year-old man presents with a three-day history of dry cough, haemoptysis and dyspnoea. He feels otherwise well. He smokes 20 cigarettes per day but there is no other relevant history.

Hb	10.6 g/dL
WBC	8.2×10^9/L
Platelets	400×10^9/L
Na	142 mmol/L
K	5.7 mmol/L
Urea	17.2 mmol/L
Creatinine	370 μmol/L
ANA	Negative
CXR	Patchy shadowing in both bases

a) What three tests would you perform to establish a diagnosis?
b) What is the likely diagnosis?

A → 222

67

5.6

A 27-year-old Asian woman presents with a six-month history of malaise, arthralgia and intermittent blurring of vision. More recently she has noticed cramp-like pains in her right arm, which are provoked by use of the arm and relieved by rest. Examination reveals an early-diastolic murmur. Her blood pressure is recorded at 170/100 in the right arm, 110/50 in the left arm and 175/100 in both legs.

ESR	60 mm/h
Rheumatoid factor	Negative
ANA	Negative
ANCA	Negative
VDRL	Negative
TPHA	Negative
CXR	Widening of aortic arch

A → 223

a) What test would you perform to establish the diagnosis?
b) What diagnosis is suggested by the above data?

5.7

A 45-year-old woman has noticed that her fingers have become puffy and itchy over the past six months. They also become intensely white and painful in cold weather.

Hb	12.5 g/dL
WBC	7.2×10^9/L
Platelets	280×10^9/L
ESR	30 mm/h
Rheumatoid factor	Positive
ANA	Positive
Anti-topoisomerase 1	Negative
Anti-centromere	Positive
Anti-RNP	Negative

A → 225

a) What diagnosis is suggested by the data?
b) What other classical features might be present or develop?
c) What further test may give characteristic changes?

RHEUMATOLOGY

5.8

A 47-year-old woman is referred for investigation of recurrent oral candidiasis. She gives a one-year history of pain and stiffness affecting the small joints of the hands and feet and a six-month history of dyspareunia. More recently she has noticed that wearing contact lenses has become uncomfortable and she finds it difficult to swallow food unless she 'washes it down' with a drink.

Hb	12.5 g/dL
WBC	3.5×10^9/L
Neutrophils	1.2×10^9/L
Platelets	280×10^9/L
ESR	50 mm/h
Rheumatoid factor	Positive
ANA	Negative
Anti-SSA	Positive
Anti-Scl-70	Negative

a) What is the likely diagnosis?
b) Name a possible cause of the haematological abnormality?
c) What additional feature of this cause would you expect to find on clinical examination?
d) What other associated condition may have arisen?
e) What three additional investigations would you perform to aid diagnosis?

A → 226

5.9

A 22-year-old army recruit presents to his medical officer complaining of dysuria and a painful, swollen right knee. One week earlier he had been off sick with diarrhoea and vomiting.

Urethral swabs	Negative	
Urine culture	Negative	
Synovial fluid	White cells	8000/ml (60% neutrophils)
	Microscopy	no organisms
		no crystals
	Culture	no growth

a) What is the most likely diagnosis?

A → 229

5.10

A 55-year-old man presents to the Accident and Emergency department with an acutely swollen left knee. He has no history of joint problems but has recently started treatment for swollen ankles.

Synovial fluid	WBC	12000/ml (80% neutrophils)
	Microscopy	no organisms
		negatively birefringent crystals present
Serum urate	410 µmol/L	(normal 180–420)

a) What is the diagnosis?
b) What treatment might he be receiving for the swollen ankles?

5.11

A worried mother takes her three-year-old son to the Accident and Emergency department with an eight-week history of spiking fevers, general malaise and reluctance to walk or play. She has also noticed a recurrent rash over his trunk and thighs. On examination the child has a pyrexia of 39°C and widespread lymphadenopathy and there is evidence of arthritis affecting the knees and elbows.

Hb	13.5 g/dL	
WBC	17.2×10^9/L	
	(80% neutrophils)	
Platelets	280×10^9/L	
ESR	45 mm/h	
CRP	32 mg/L	(normal < 10)
Rheumatoid factor	Negative	
ANA	Negative	
ANCA	Negative	
Urine dipstick	Blood	negative
	Protein	trace
Blood culture (× 3)	Negative	
Urine culture	Negative	
Throat swab	Negative	
ASOT	60 U/ml	(normal < 200)

a) What is the likely diagnosis?

RHEUMATOLOGY

5.12

A 12-year-old Jewish boy presents to the Accident and Emergency department with a six-hour history of severe abdominal pain accompanied by a painful swollen right knee. He has a pyrexia of 39.1°C and on examination of his abdomen there is marked rebound tenderness and guarding. He has been admitted with similar symptoms on three previous occasions in the past year but has been well between attacks. On the last occasion he also developed severe pleuritic chest pain. VQ scan was normal. One of his younger cousins has also recently had a similar attack.

Hb	13.1 g/dL	
WBC	16.4×10^9/L	(78% neutrophils)
Platelets	350×10^9/L	
ESR	55 mm/hour	
ANA	Negative	
Urine dipstick	Blood	negative
	Protein	negative
Synovial fluid	White cells	10000/ml (60% neutrophils)
	Microscopy	no organisms
		no crystals
	Culture	no growth

a) What is the most likely diagnosis?
b) What is the major complication of this condition?
c) After the acute episode what treatment is indicated?

A → 233

6 NEUROLOGY

NEUROLOGY

6.1

A 28-year-old man is admitted with a two-day history of vague headache and lethargy. Over the past 12 h he has become increasingly drowsy. On examination he has a pyrexia of 38.4°C but there is no neck stiffness and no rash.

Glucose	5.3 mmol/L	
Lumbar puncture	Opening pressure	28 cm CSF
	Red cells	10/ml
	White cells	200/ml (85% polymorphs)
	Protein	1.92 g/L
	Glucose	2.2 mmol/L

a) What is the diagnosis?
b) What is your immediate treatment?

A → 235

6.2

A 35-year-old woman presents with a 72-h history of increasing confusion. On examination she is drowsy with mild right-sided weakness and a positive Babinski sign on the right. She also has a right-sided, upper quadrantic hemianopia. Of note: her husband said that two days previously she had repeatedly mentioned that she could smell fresh coffee.

Glucose	6.3 mmol/L	
Lumbar puncture	Opening pressure	35 cm CSF
	Red cells	2/ml
	White cells	70/ml (70% lymphocytes)
	Protein	1.1 g/L
	Glucose	2.2 mmol/L
	Gram stain	no organisms

a) Name the two most likely differential diagnoses.
b) Name three further investigations.

A → 236

6.3

A 19-year-old student is admitted for investigation of headache and general malaise of three weeks' duration. On examination she has moderate neck stiffness, weakness of abduction of the left eye and asymmetry of facial movements.

Na	128 mmol/L		
K	3.8 mmol/L		
Urea	8.1 mmol/L		
Glucose	6.6 mmol/L		
Lumbar puncture	Red cells	12/ml	
	White cells	110/ml	(66% lymphocytes, 30% polymorphs)
	Protein	1.8 g/L	
	Glucose	2.6 mmol/L	

a) What is the diagnosis?
b) What complication may have developed?

6.4

A 58-year-old man is referred to the neurologist for investigation of poor memory and uncharacteristic behaviour of recent onset. On examination he is noted to have poor concentration and intermittent myoclonus. Mini mental test score = 5/10.

Glucose	5.5 mmol/L		
Lumbar puncture	Red cells	3/ml	
	White cells	3/ml	(lymphocytes)
	Protein	0.3 g/L	
	Glucose	4.2 mmol/L	
CT brain	Cerebral atrophy		
EEG	Periodic biphasic sharp waveforms		

a) What is the diagnosis?

6.5

A seven-year-old boy presents to the GP with a sore throat, earache and severe headache. The GP diagnoses tonsillitis and prescribes amoxycillin. Twelve hours later the patient is admitted to casualty following a grand-mal seizure.

Glucose	4.5 mmol/L		
Lumbar puncture	Red cells	50/ml	
	White cells	150/ml	(60% lymphocytes, 30% polymorphs)
	Protein	2.1 g/L	
	Glucose	1.2 mmol/L	
	Gram stain	no organisms seen	

a) What is the diagnosis?
b) What is the main differential diagnosis?

A → 238

6.6

A 30-year-old woman presents with severe headache. She gives a five-week history of 'heaviness' of the legs. On examination she has weakness of abduction of the left eye and bilaterally upward-going plantar responses. Reflexes in the legs are brisk but those in the arms are normal.

Glucose	5.5 mmol/L		
Lumbar puncture	Red cells	10/ml	
	White cells	4/ml	(lymphocytes)
	Protein	4.1 g/L	
	Glucose	3.2 mmol/L	
	Gram stain	no organisms seen	
CT brain	Dilation of the lateral ventricles. No other abnormalities seen.		

a) What is the most likely diagnosis?
b) What investigation would you perform to confirm this diagnosis?
c) What is the cause of the dilated ventricles?

A → 239

6.7

A 56-year-old woman is referred for investigation of intermittent diplopia. Further questioning reveals that she often has difficulty with chewing and swallowing towards the end of a large meal.

Hb	9.8g/dL
WCC	4.2×10^9/L
Platelets	120×10^9/L
MCV	110fL
CT brain	Normal
EMG	Progressive reduction in amplitude of evoked potentials with repetitive stimulation

a) What is the cause of the abnormal neurology?
b) What is the probable haematological diagnosis?
c) What investigation would you perform to confirm the neurological diagnosis?
d) Name two further investigations that are appropriate.

A → 240

6.8

A 60-year-old man has noticed increasing difficulty in climbing stairs. On examination he has bilateral wasting of the quadriceps and an erythematous rash affecting the face and forearms. There are also raised erythematous papules over the knuckles and proximal interphalangeal joints.

ESR	55mm/h
Rheumatoid factor	Positive
ANA	Positive
ANCA	Negative
EMG	Short duration polyphasic potentials, spontaneous fibrillation and high frequency repetitive discharges

a) What is the likely diagnosis?
b) What two additional investigations would you perform to confirm the diagnosis?

A → 241

NEUROLOGY

6.9

A 25-year-old college student is referred to the neurologist for investigation of double vision. On examination she has impaired abduction of the left eye, nystagmus and mild ataxia. The results of her visual evoked potentials (VEPs) are shown below.

a) What abnormality is present in the VEPs?
b) What is the most likely diagnosis?
c) What additional test would you perform to confirm the diagnosis?

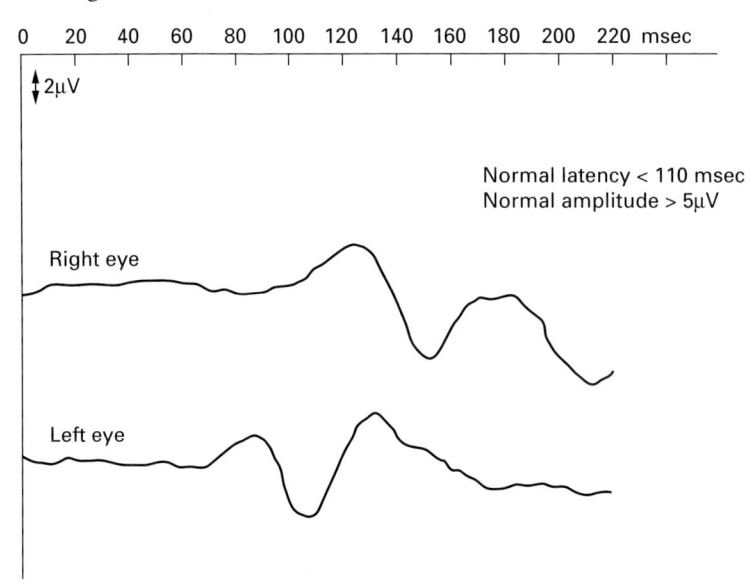

A → 242

```
0   20   40   60   80   100   120   140   160   180   200   220  msec
```

↕ 2µV

Normal latency < 110 msec
Normal amplitude > 5µV

Right eye

Left eye

Fig. 6.1

6.10

A 55-year-old woman has noticed tingling in the fingers of her right hand and slightly reduced dexterity. Below are the results of nerve conduction studies for the median nerve.

a) What is the conduction velocity distal to stimulus 2?
b) What is the conduction velocity from the elbow to wrist?
c) What is the diagnosis?

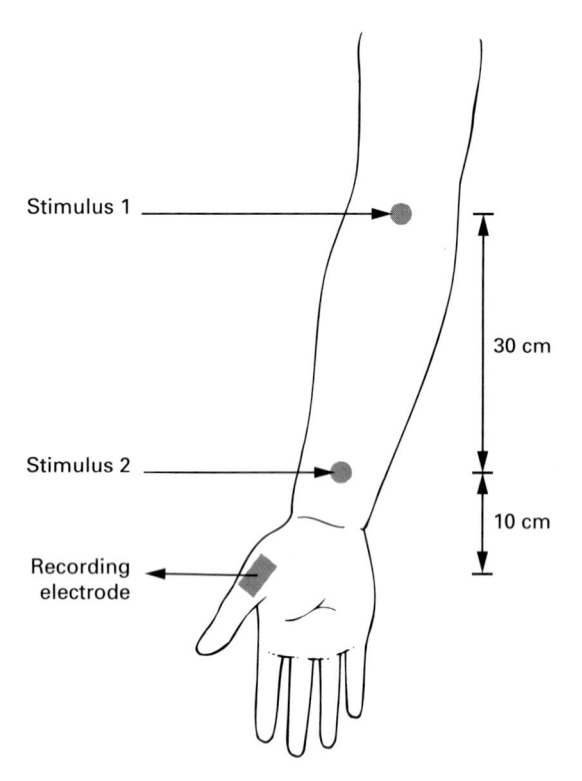

A → 244

Stimulus 1

30 cm

Stimulus 2

10 cm

Recording electrode

Latency of response following stimulus 1 = 7.7 msec
Latency of response following stimulus 2 = 2.7 msec

Fig. 6.2

NEUROLOGY

6.11

These are the results of nerve conduction studies performed on a 21-year-old woman.

Sural nerve (sensory)		
Conduction velocity	44 msec^{-1}	(normal > 50)
Amplitude	2 mV	(normal > 17)
Anterior tibial nerve (motor)		
Conduction velocity	47 msec^{-1}	(normal > 45)
Amplitude	21 mV	(normal > 20)

a) What abnormality is present?
b) Suggest two causes.

A → 244

6.12

Below is the pure tone audiogram of a 55-year-old woman who is being investigated for attacks of vertigo. She has also noticed troublesome right-sided tinnitus.

a) What abnormality does the audiogram show?
b) What is the likely diagnosis?

A → 246

○ Air conduction
● Bone conduction

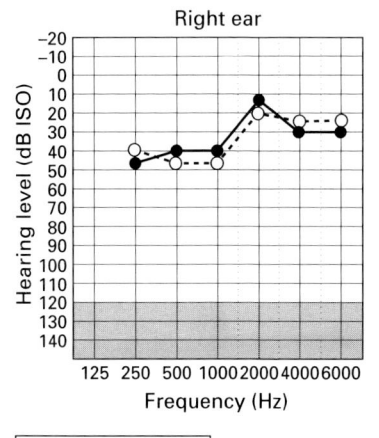

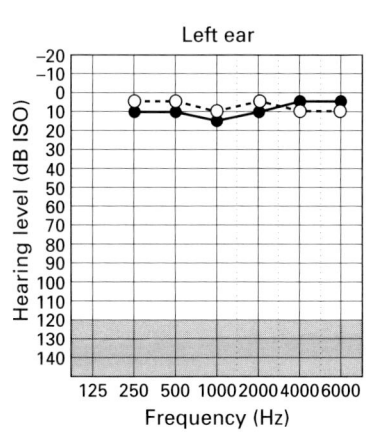

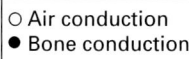

Fig. 6.3

6.13

Below is the pure tone audiogram of a 35-year-old soldier who is being investigated for unilateral tinnitus.

a) What is the most likely cause of this abnormality?

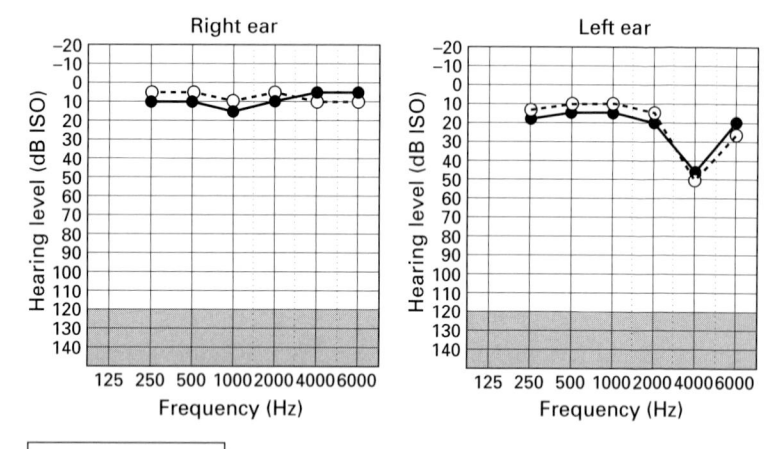

A → 246

Fig. 6.4

6.14

Below is the pure tone audiogram of 66-year-old woman who presented to her GP with worsening hearing loss of three months' duration.

a) What abnormality does it show?
b) What is the most likely diagnosis?

A → 247

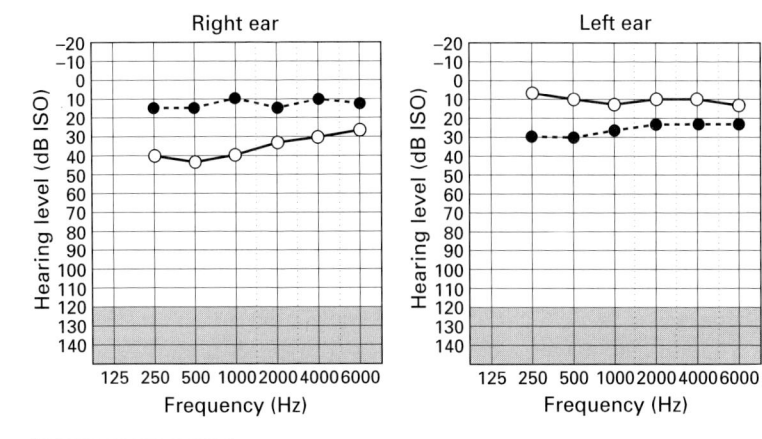

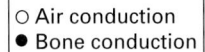

Fig. 6.5

6.15

A 45-year-old man presents with unsteadiness. On examination he has nystagmus with a fast phase to the right side and an absent corneal reflex on the left. His pure tone audiogram is shown below.

a) What investigation is indicated?
b) What is the likely diagnosis?

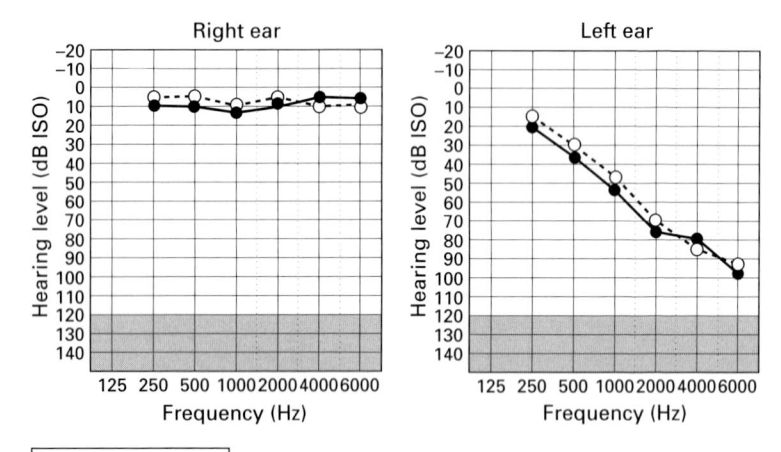

A → 247

Right ear / Left ear audiogram

○ Air conduction
● Bone conduction

Fig. 6.6

6.16

Below is the pure tone audiogram of a 40-year-old man who complains of progressive hearing loss over the past two years.

a) What is the diagnosis?

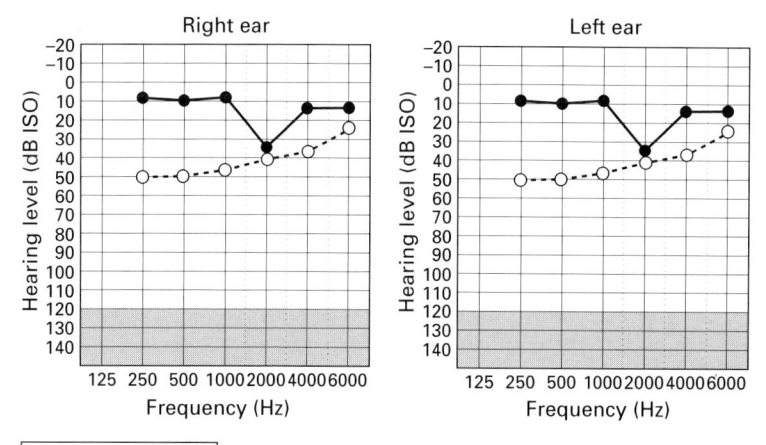

A → 248

Fig. 6.7

○ Air conduction
● Bone conduction

83

7 RESPIRATORY MEDICINE

RESPIRATORY MEDICINE

7.1

Below is the spirometry trace from a 45-year-old man who has been referred to the chest clinic for investigation of nocturnal cough.

a) What is the FEV_1?
b) What is the FVC?
c) Name a probable cause of the nocturnal cough.
d) What additional test would you perform?

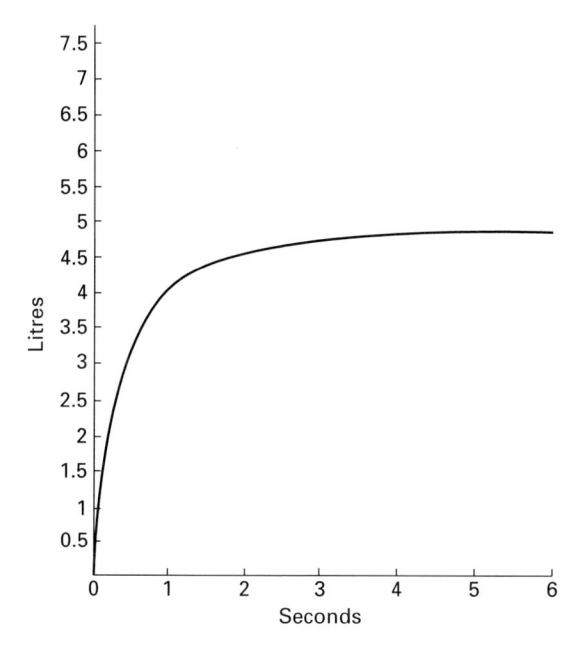

A → 253

Fig. 7.1

85

7.2

Below is the flow volume curve of a 50-year-old man who is being investigated for shortness of breath.

a) What two differential diagnoses does the flow volume curve suggest?
b) How might you distinguish between them?

A → 254

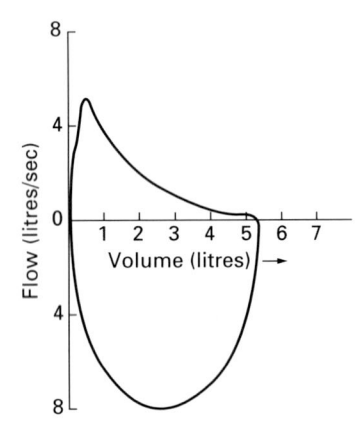

Fig. 7.2

7.3

A 58-year-old man is under investigation by haematologists for an abnormality on his blood film. Lung function tests are subsequently performed for investigation of a transient episode of pleuritic chest pain associated with shortness of breath.

	Actual	Predicted	% Predicted
FEV_1 (L)	3.7	3.86	95
FVC (L)	4.95	4.87	101
FEV_1/FVC (%)	74	79	
V_A (L)	6.9	6.8	101
T_LCO (mmol/min/kPa)	13.5	9.8	137
KCO (mmol/min/kPa/L)	1.96	1.52	129

a) What is the likely abnormality on the blood film?
b) What is the likely diagnosis?
c) What was the likely cause of the pleuritic chest pain?
d) What other conditions may cause this abnormality of lung function?

A → 254

7.4

Below is the flow volume curve of a patient who presents with a two-year history of dry cough. He takes indomethacin for chronic low back pain.

a) What pattern of abnormality does it show?
b) Name two possible contributory factors.
c) What is the unifying diagnosis?

A → 255

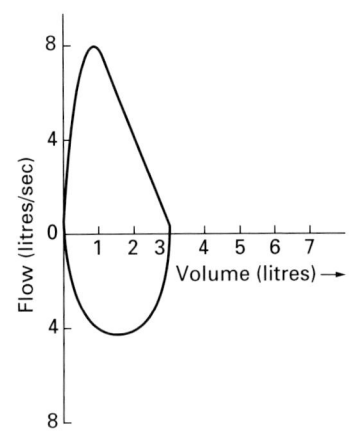

Fig. 7.3

7.5

A 55-year-old miner has noticed that he is considerably more short of breath than usual when out walking his dog. His symptoms are particularly noticeable on climbing the short incline back to his house. His lung function tests are as follows.

	Actual	Predicted	% Predicted
FEV_1 (L)	1.23	3.09	40
FVC (L)	2.37	3.96	60
FEV_1/FVC (%)	52	78	67
RV (L)	5.69	2.57	221
V_A (L)	3.8	7.2	53
T_LCO (mmol/min/kPa)	8.53	7.05	121

a) Describe the abnormalities present on lung function.
b) What is the diagnosis?

A → 256

7.6

A 45-year-old man is admitted to hospital with progressive difficulty walking and mild shortness of breath on exertion. On examination tendon reflexes are absent and there is marked proximal muscle weakness. Ten days earlier he received a course of ciprofloxacin for a diarrhoeal illness from which he has now recovered. Below is the result of spirometry performed on the day of admission.

a) Name a likely diagnosis.
b) What further investigations would you perform?
c) What urgent treatment may be necessary?

A → 256

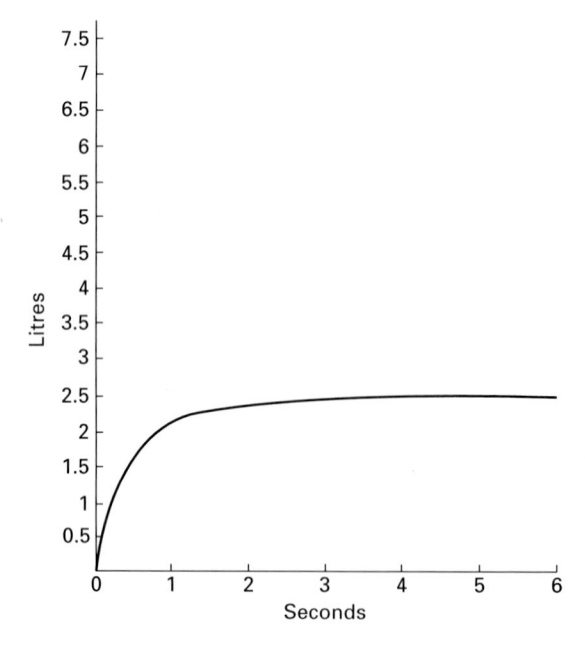

Fig. 7.4

RESPIRATORY MEDICINE

7.7

A 40-year-old man presents with a history of increasing shortness of breath over several months and more recent onset of an erythematous rash affecting his lower legs. He has also had two episodes of haemoptysis. His PMH consists only of asthma. He does not smoke and is not on medication. Chest X-ray shows an area of ill-defined shadowing at the right base and similar areas in the left mid-zone. Blood, urine and lung function tests are shown below.

	Actual	Predicted	% Predicted
FEV_1 (L)	3.82	3.75	101
FVC (L)	4.75	4.80	99
FEV_1/FVC (%)	80	78	
T_LCO (mmol/min/kPa)	12.7	9.5	134
Hb	14.3g/dL		
WCC	11.6×10^9/L	(16% eosinophils)	
Platelets	350×10^9/L		
Urine dipstick	+++ positive for red blood cells		

a) What is the likely diagnosis?
b) Name two other possible diagnoses.
c) What three further investigations would you perform?

A → 257

7.8

Below is the flow volume curve of a 48-year-old woman who is being investigated for chronic cough and shortness of breath on exertion.

a) What abnormality does the curve suggest?
b) What would be your next course of action?

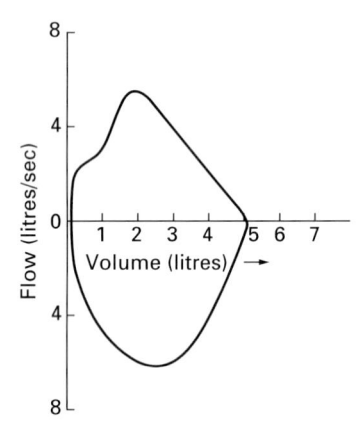

Fig. 7.5

7.9

A 27-year-old man has been referred to the respiratory clinic for assessment of gradually worsening difficulty in breathing that is more pronounced on lying flat and partially relieved by sitting upright. The only past medical history is that of a prolonged period of recovery following a childhood illness. His lung function tests are as follows.

	Actual	Predicted	% Predicted
FEV_1 (L)	2.22	4.0	55
FVC (L)	3.02	4.64	65
FEV_1/FVC (%)	74	79	
T_LCO (mmol/min/kPa)	7.24	10.16	71
KCO (mmol/min/kPa/L)	1.73	1.51	115

a) What abnormality of lung function is shown?
b) What is the likely cause?
c) What was the childhood illness?

RESPIRATORY MEDICINE

7.10

Below is the flow volume loop of a 55-year-old man who six months earlier had spent one month in the intensive care unit where he required prolonged mechanical ventilation following injury in a car accident.

a) What complication does the flow volume loop suggest?

A → 260

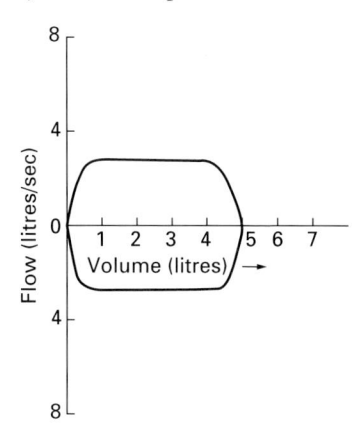

Fig. 7.6

7.11

A 35-year-old woman is being investigated for severe breathlessness of six months' duration. She does not smoke and has had no previous illnesses. Her only medication is the oral contraceptive pill. Her Hb = 12.3 g/dL. Her lung function is shown below.

	Actual	Predicted	% Predicted
FEV_1 (L)	2.9	2.85	102
FVC (L)	3.40	3.3	103
FEV_1/FVC (%)	85	79	
V_A (L)	6.15	9.4	98
T_LCO (mmol/min/kPa)	6.11	6.3	65

a) What is the likely diagnosis?
b) Name two other causes of this abnormality of lung function.

A → 261

7.12

Below is the flow volume loop of a 27-year-old woman who is being investigated for reduced exercise tolerance and raised liver enzymes. She is a non-smoker.

a) What lung condition does the flow volume loop suggest?
b) What test would you perform to establish the underlying cause?

A → 262

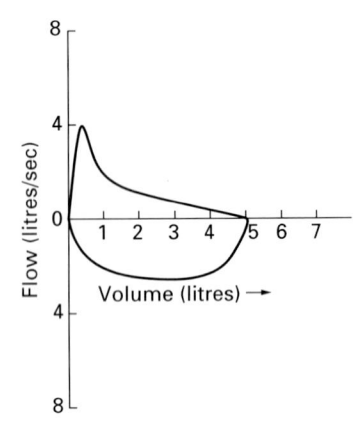

Fig. 7.7

7.13

A 28-year-old woman has been referred by her GP for investigation of a chronic cough. She has also begun to wake up short of breath at night. Her lung function is shown below.

	Actual	Predicted	% Predicted
FEV_1 (L)	1.85	2.46	75
FVC (L)	3.01	3.38	89
FEV_1/FVC (%)	62	79	79
T_LCO (mmol/min/kPa)	10.92	8.7	116
KCO (mmol/min/kPa/L)	2.20	1.52	145

A → 262

a) What is the most likely diagnosis?

8 GASTROENTEROLOGY

8.1

A 55-year-old man is being investigated for weight loss, recurrent central abdominal pain and intermittent diarrhoea.

Hb	12.1 g/dL	
MCV	101	
Calcium	1.80 mmol/L	
Phosphate	0.78 mmol/L	
Albumin	28 g/L	
Bilirubin	13 µmol/L	(normal < 17)
AST	50 IU/L	(normal 13–42)
ALP	160 IU/L	(normal 40–115)
Gamma GT	80 IU/L	(normal < 40)
B_{12} and folate	Normal	
Faecal fat	55 mmol/24h	(normal < 18)

a) What is the cause of the low calcium?
b) What is the cause of the low phosphate?
c) What is the most likely diagnosis?
d) What is the most likely cause?

8.2

A six-year-old boy is being investigated for failure to thrive. He has a history of recurrent chest infections and his GP has recently diagnosed asthma.

| Faecal fat | 55 mmol/24h (normal < 18) |
| Oral D-xylose (25g) absorption test: | 4g excreted after 5h |

a) What does the D-xylose absorption test demonstrate?
b) What is the likely diagnosis?
c) How would you confirm this?
d) What three further tests would you perform?
e) After appropriate treatment name one further appropriate course of action.

8.3

A 45-year-old sergeant in the Royal Fusiliers, who has recently returned from Bosnia, is referred for investigation of three months of diarrhoea and weight loss. He has been in the army for 20 years and served for many years in India, until about five years ago. His only medical history is of surgery for a gastric ulcer six years earlier.

Hb	9.8 g/dL	
WCC	5.4×10^9/L	
Platelets	188×10^9/L	
MCV	103 fL	
Faecal fat	55 mmol/24 h	(normal < 18)

a) Name four possible diagnoses.
b) Name four appropriate investigations.

A → 267

8.4

A 35-year-old labourer is being investigated for abdominal bloating and weight loss. He is noted to have a pruritic vesicular rash.

Hb	10.1 g/dL	
WCC	6.1 × 10⁹/L	
Platelets	121 × 10⁹/L	
MCV	102 fL	
RDW	17%	(normal 13.2 +/− 1.6%)
Blood film	Macrocytes, target cells and Howell–Jolly bodies	
Ferritin	210 µg/L	(normal < 300)
Na	138 mmol/L	
K	4.1 mmol/L	
Urea	6.7 mmol/L	
Glucose	5.6 mmol/L	
Bicarbonate	27 mmol/L	
Calcium	1.71 mmol/L	
Phosphate	0.68 mmol/L	
Albumin	28 g/L	
Bilirubin	18 µmol/L	(normal < 17)
AST	30 IU/L	(normal 13–42)
ALP	190 IU/L	(normal 40–115)

a) What is the diagnosis?
b) Name three appropriate investigations.
c) How do you explain the blood film?
d) What is the rash?
e) What is the treatment?

A → 268

GASTROENTEROLOGY

8.5

A 60-year-old Asian woman is referred by her GP with low back pain.

Hb	10.2 g/dL	
WCC	6.7×10^9/L	
Platelets	233×10^9/L	
MCV	109 fL	
Calcium	2.01 mmol/L	
Phosphate	0.82 mmol/L	
Albumin	38 g/L	
ALP	160 IU/L	(normal 40–115)
Faecal fat	12 mmol/24 h	(normal < 18)

a) What is the likely diagnosis?
b) What is the cause of the low back pain?
c) Why might she find it difficult to climb stairs?

A → 269

8.6

A 55-year-old Asian woman is being investigated for macrocytic anaemia.

Faecal fat	30 mmol/24 h	(normal < 18)
Schilling test		
^{58}Co-B$_{12}$ alone	4% of dose excreted at 24 h	
^{58}Co-B$_{12}$ + intrinsic factor	5% of dose excreted at 24 h	
(^{14}C) glycocholic acid breath test	level in breath peaks at 2 h	

a) What is the likely diagnosis?
b) Name three predisposing conditions.
c) What test could you perform to confirm your diagnosis?

A → 270

8.7

A 35-year-old man is admitted as an emergency with acute appendicitis. Twenty-four hours after appendicectomy his blood tests are as follows.

Hb	12.2 g/dL	
Reticulocytes	1.5%	
Haptoglobin	2.2 g/L	(normal 0.6–2.6)
Albumin	38 g/L	
Bilirubin	67 µmol/L	(normal < 17)
AST	30 IU/L	(normal 13–42)
ALP	101 IU/L	(normal 40–115)
Urine dipstick	Negative to bilirubin	

a) What is the most likely diagnosis?
b) What two investigations would you do to confirm the diagnosis?

A → 272

8.8

These are the results of a 50-year-old woman who has intractable pruritus.

Albumin	30 g/L	
Bilirubin	70 µmol/L	(normal < 17)
AST	50 IU/L	(normal 13–42)
ALP	550 IU/L	(normal 40–115)
IgA	1.6 g/L	(normal 0.8–4.0)
IgG	10.0 g/L	(normal 5.3–16.5)
IgM	5.2 g/L	(normal 0.5–2.0)
Caeruloplasmin	500 mg/L	(normal 200–400)
Liver biopsy reveals increased copper content (in addition to histological changes)		

a) What diagnosis is suggested by the above results?
b) What two investigations would you do to confirm the diagnosis?
c) What histological features may be seen?

A → 273

8.9

A 24-year-old woman with no past medical history was found to have abnormal liver function by her GP. He diagnosed hepatitis A infection and reassured her. Eight months later her liver function is as shown below. There is no history of alcohol abuse.

Albumin	30 g/L	
Bilirubin	90 μmol/L	(normal < 17)
AST	450 IU/L	(normal 13–42)
ALP	198 IU/L	(normal 40–115)
IgA	5.6 g/L	(normal 0.8–4.0)
IgG	30.0 g/L	(normal 5.3–16.5)
IgM	2.4 g/L	(normal 0.5–2.0)
Hep B SAg	Negative	

a) What is the most likely diagnosis?
b) List five differential diagnoses.
c) What histological change will the liver biopsy show?
d) What five further investigations would you do?

A → 274

8.10

A 55-year-old man is referred to a gastroenterologist for investigation of weight loss and diarrhoea. He gives a two-year history of intermittent arthritis of the right knee and ankle and has recently been diagnosed as suffering from epilepsy.

Anti-gliadin antibodies	-ve
Anti-endomysial antibodies	-ve
Faecal fat	52 mmol/24 h (normal < 18)
Stool microscopy	No intestinal parasites, cysts or ova
Jejunal biopsy	Villi are blunted and the lamina propria contains a dense infiltrate of macrophages that stain strongly with periodic acid-Schiff (PAS)

a) What is the diagnosis?
b) What is the treatment?

A → 275

99

8.11

A 56-year-old man presents to the Accident and Emergency department with prolonged bleeding following a dental extraction. Examination reveals a well-tanned man with a 2 cm hepatomegaly and several spider naevi. His past medical history consists only of several episodes of gout affecting the right knee and he is not on medication.

Hb	14.5 g/dL	
WCC	9.1 × 10⁹/L	
Platelets	87 × 10⁹/L	
Na	138 mmol/L	
K	4.1 mmol/L	
Urea	9.1 mmol/L	
Creatinine	130 µmol/L	
Glucose	13.1 mmol/L	
Albumin	30 g/L	
Bilirubin	25 µmol/L	(normal < 17)
AST	80 IU/L	(normal 13–42)
ALP	150 IU/L	(normal 40–115)

a) What is the likely diagnosis?
b) Give three investigations to confirm it.
c) Name three other investigations.
d) Give two reasons why this man might be impotent.

A → 276

PART 2

ANSWERS

1 CARDIOLOGY

CARDIOLOGY

CARDIAC CATHETERIZATION

Table 1.1 Indices that can be directly measured or calculated during cardiac catheterization

	Normal values (mmHg unless stated otherwise)
1. Left-sided catheterization	
• Aortic pressures	120/80 (mean = 95)
• LV pressures (end-systolic/end-diastolic)	150/5–10
• Oxygen saturation (aorta, LV, LA)	98%
2. Right-sided catheterization	
• IVC/SVC pressure	
• RA pressures	0–8 (mean)
• RV pressures (end-systolic/end-diastolic)	15–30/0–8
• PA pressures (end-systolic/end-diastolic)	15–30/3–12 (mean = 9–16)
• PCWP (closely approximates LA pressure)	1–10 (mean)
• Oxygen saturation (vena cava, RA, RV, PA)	74% (SVC ~ 70%)
3. LV cineangiography	
• Calculation of LV end-diastolic (LVEDV) and end-systolic (LVESV) volumes	
NB: *The algorithm assumes that LV is an ellipse*	
• Calculation of stroke volume (SV = LVEDV − LVESV)	40–70 ml/m^2
• Calculation of ejection fraction (EF = SV/LVEDV)	
• Calculation of LV mass	
• Assessment of regional wall motion	
• Assessment of MV competence	
4. Selective angiography of coronary arteries	
5. Calculation of cardiac output	2.8–4.2 L/min/m^2
6. Calculation of systemic and pulmonary vascular resistance	
7. Calculation of cardiac work	

1.1

a) The oxygen saturation in the superior vena cava (SVC) and right atrium (RA) should be approximately the same. The observed 'step-up' in saturation between the SVC and RA indicates that there must be an abnormal connection between the two sides of the heart, at the level of the atria, with left to right shunting of blood, that is, an atrial septal defect (ASD). Partial anomalous pulmonary venous drainage can produce a similar step-up in saturation if the anomalous veins drain directly into the RA, but this condition is usually associated with mild central cyanosis.

b) Complications may include pulmonary hypertension, Eisenmenger complex (see answer to Q 1.5), supraventricular arrhythmias and paradoxical emboli.

c) Right bundle branch block (RBBB) and right axis deviation are characteristic of ostium secundum ASDs, whereas RBBB and left axis deviation are characteristically seen in ostium primum ASDs. This patient still has normal pulmonary artery pressures at the age of 20 and is therefore most likely to have an ostium secundum ASD. Ostium primum ASDs lie just above the atrioventricular valves and extend into the anterior leaflet of the mitral valve producing mitral regurgitation, which increases the left to right shunt resulting in earlier onset of symptoms and a worse prognosis.

d) The treatment of choice is surgical (or device) closure since the patient is young and pulmonary hypertension has not yet developed.

1.2

a) The pressures in the femoral artery approximate to those of the aorta, and the systolic pressure in the aorta should be approximately the same as in the left ventricle (LV). The data show a systolic pressure gradient between the LV and the femoral artery. Since the aortic pressure is not given, this may represent a pressure gradient across the aortic valve, that is, aortic stenosis, or a pressure gradient across an obstruction in the aorta itself, such as in coarctation of the aorta. In this case, however, the high pressure in the femoral artery makes coarctation unlikely.

b) At 45 years of age there is a reasonable chance that this patient may have co-existing coronary artery disease contributing to his symptoms. Angiography of the coronary arteries is therefore required prior to valve replacement so that diseased arteries can be treated with bypass grafting at the same operation.

c) Conventional wisdom states that the valve should be replaced when the pressure gradient is > 50 mm Hg. The pressure gradient in this patient is only 42 mm Hg but he is already symptomatic. Since the prognosis with conservative treatment is considerably worse once aortic stenosis has become symptomatic this patient should be referred for aortic valve replacement.

1.3

a) There is a 'step-up' in oxygen saturation between the right atrium (RA) and right ventricle (RV) indicating that there must be an abnormal connection between the two sides of the heart, at the level of the ventricles, with left to right shunting of blood, that is a ventricular septal defect (VSD). The pulmonary artery pressure is also high, indicating that pulmonary hypertension has developed.

b) Surgical closure of the defect.

VSD is the most common congenital cardiac abnormality but acquired septal defects can occur after myocardial infarction. The abnormal connection between the ventricles allows left to right shunting of blood, which increases pulmonary blood flow and may result in pulmonary hypertension (because of obliterative vascular changes) and Eisenmenger syndrome (see answer to Q 1.5). Most congenital defects occur in the membranous part of the septum rather than in the muscular part, but there are numerous sites at which the defect can occur and the natural history is therefore dependent upon both the site and the size of the defect.

Small VSDs (*Maladie de Roger*) need no treatment (unless symptomatic or endocarditis develops), as they tend to close spontaneously with time. Larger VSDs (pulmonary:systemic flow ratio greater than 3:1) and those causing symptoms or elevated pulmonary pressures (such as in this patient) require surgical closure before irreversible pulmonary hypertension develops. Because of the risk of bacterial endocarditis all patients with VSD require antibiotic prophylaxis for any procedure that may result in bacteraemia, for example dental procedures, urinary catheterization, obstetric/gynaecological procedures, surgery/instrumentation of the lower bowel and so on.

1.4

a) There is an elevated left atrial (LA) pressure with normal left ventricular (LV) pressures. Although only the mean left atrial pressure is given, there will almost certainly be an end-diastolic pressure gradient between the LA and LV. This indicates that mitral stenosis is present. If the symptoms of left heart failure were caused by LV dysfunction, diastolic dysfunction or mitral regurgitation, then one would expect the LV end-diastolic pressure to be elevated. The most common cause of mitral stenosis is rheumatic heart disease.

b) The pulmonary artery (PA) and right ventricular (RV) pressures are elevated indicating that pulmonary hypertension and right ventricular hypertrophy have developed.

c) Atrial fibrillation and systemic emboli (cerebral, pulmonary, coronary, splenic, mesenteric or renal; the arteries of the limbs are most commonly affected) may also complicate mitral stenosis.

d) Conservative treatment is no longer appropriate as severe symptoms have developed. The choice of treatment therefore lies between valvuloplasty, mitral valvotomy, or valve replacement and anticoagulation. The nature of this patient's symptoms indicate severe mitral stenosis and valve replacement will therefore probably be necessary.

1.5

a) The oxygen saturation in the femoral vein should be approximately the same as that of the right atrium. The data shows a step-up in saturation between the femoral vein and the right atrium, which indicates the presence of a left to right shunt somewhere between these two points. This is only anatomically feasible at the level of the atrium, that is an atrial septal defect.

b) The patient has developed severe pulmonary hypertension with reversal of the direction of shunting of blood (shunt reversal). Consequently, deoxygenated blood is shunted from the RA to the LA producing low left-sided oxygen saturations and cyanosis – this is the Eisenmenger reaction and Eisenmenger complex has developed.

CARDIOLOGY Ⓐ

1.6

a) There is a pressure gradient between the right ventricle and the pulmonary artery indicating that pulmonary stenosis is present. There is also a step-down in oxygen saturation between the left atrium and the left ventricle indicating that there is an abnormal connection between the two sides of the heart at the level of the ventricles, that is a ventricular septal defect (VSD) with right to left shunting of blood. In addition there is a step-down in oxygen saturation at the level of the aorta. This could theoretically be caused by a patent ductus arteriosus with right to left shunting of blood. In view of the other abnormalities, however, it is more likely to represent an 'over-riding aorta' (blood from both the RV and the LV exits through the aorta), with this combination of abnormalities then comprising Fallot's tetralogy.

b) Fallot's tetralogy.

c) The lung fields will appear oligaemic as a result of pulmonary stenosis.

Fallot's tetralogy

This accounts for about 10% of all congenital heart lesions and is the commonest cause of cyanotic disease presenting after one year of age. The four characteristic abnormalities that combine to form Fallot's tetralogy are:

1. Ventricular septal defect.
2. Right ventricular outflow obstruction – the level of the obstruction is most commonly infundibular (50%) but may also be valvular, supravalvular or a combination.
3. Over-riding aorta – the aorta lies directly over the VSD so that blood from both the right and left ventricle exits through it.
4. Right ventricular hypertrophy.

Surgical correction of the abnormalities is the ideal treatment but very young infants and those with polycythaemia greater than 21 g/dl of haemoglobin may be treated with a shunt procedure initially (e.g. Blalock–Taussig shunt).

1.7

a) There is a step-up in oxygen saturation between the right ventricle (RV) and the pulmonary artery (PA) indicating the presence of an abnormal connection between the pulmonary and systemic circulations, with left to right shunting of blood, at the level of the pulmonary artery. The most likely cause is a patent ductus arteriosus (PDA).

b) The patient has presented with high fever, which may be indicative of infective endocarditis. In addition the PA pressure is elevated indicating that pulmonary hypertension is developing.

c) There is a characteristic, continuous murmur that is best heard below the left clavicle in the first intercostal space or over the first rib. This murmur is caused by continuous shunting of blood from the aorta to the PA throughout both systole and diastole and it is said to sound 'machine-like'. There may also be an early diastolic murmur, heard best in the pulmonary area, caused by pulmonary regurgitation. Treatment is with surgical or device closure.

THE ELECTROCARDIOGRAM

To interpret ECG findings successfully, some definitions and characteristics of the normal ECG have to be borne in mind.

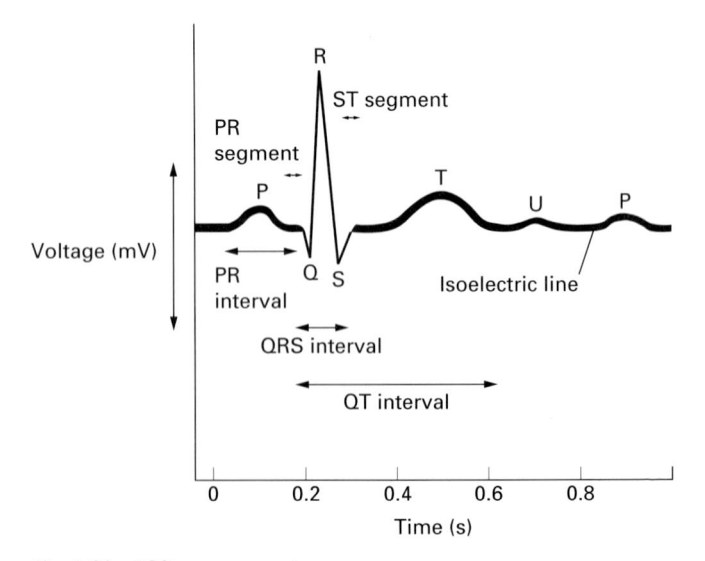

Fig. 1.20 ECG measurements

CARDIOLOGY

Table 1.2 Characteristics of normal ECG

ECG feature	Characteristics
P wave (atrial impulse)	• Normally only inverted in lead aVR
PR interval (delay in AV node)	• Measured from onset of P wave to onset of QRS complex • Normal duration 0.12–0.21s (roughly 3–5 small squares on ECG)
QRS complex (corresponds to ventricular systole)	• Normal duration < 0.1s (just under three small squares on ECG)
T wave (corresponds to ventricular repolarization)	
QT interval	• Measured from start of QRS to end of T wave • Duration varies with heart rate therefore usually corrected (QT_c) by dividing by square root of cycle length (R–R interval) $QT_c = QT / \sqrt{(R-R)}$ QT_c normally < 0.42 s
U wave	• Deflection immediately following T wave • Normal variant (? Caused by repolarization of conducting tissue) • May be prominent in hypokalaemia

1.8

a) Wolff–Parkinson–White (WPW) syndrome type A.

b) Adenosine.

Wolff–Parkinson–White syndrome

WPW is one of the pre-excitation syndromes (the other main pre-excitation syndrome being Lown–Ganong–Levine syndrome). It is characterized by a short PR interval and widened QRS complex, caused by the presence of a delta wave, together with paroxysmal tachycardia.

In WPW there is an 'accessory pathway' (the bundle of Kent) between the atria and the ventricles. Since, unlike the AV node, this accessory pathway does not delay conduction the ventricles become activated via this route before the atrial impulse has traversed the AV node. This 'pre-excitation' results in a short PR interval. The accessory pathway is not connected to specialized conducting tissue and the early part of ventricular activation is therefore slow, producing a more gradual gradient ('slurring') to the initial part of the QRS complex. This is the delta wave. Subsequent parts of the QRS complex are caused by activation of the ventricle by the slower impulse from the AV node and proceed normally. WPW is classified as type A or type B depending upon the direction of the QRS complex in lead V1. In type A WPW the accessory pathway connects to the left ventricle and the QRS complex is predominantly positive in V1. In type B WPW the accessory pathway connects to the right ventricle and the QRS is predominantly negative in lead V1.

The presence of an abnormal connection between the atria and ventricles predisposes to paroxysmal arrhythmias (approximately two-thirds of those with WPW will suffer arrhythmias), mainly atrioventricular re-entrant tachycardia and, less commonly, atrial fibrillation (AF). The former is a nuisance but the latter may be life threatening since 1:1 transmission of atrial impulses to the ventricles may occur resulting in ventricular rates of 300 bpm. Such high ventricular rates frequently degenerate into ventricular fibrillation.

Patients with symptomatic WPW should undergo electrophysiological study in order to assess the risk of pre-excited AF. This involves assessment of the refractory period of the accessory pathway and ventricular rate during induced AF. A long refractory period is associated with a low risk of pre-excited AF. These low-risk patients can be treated with drug prophylaxis although digoxin and verapamil should be avoided since they may increase the rate of conduction down the accessory pathway in the event of AF. Drugs that act on the accessory pathway are most effective (flecainide, procainamide, sotalol and amiodarone). In high-risk patients, or those with frequent troublesome arrhythmias, the treatment of choice is radiofrequency ablation of the accessory pathway(s). There is a risk of damage to the AV node and subsequent complete heart block with this procedure, particularly if the accessory pathway is close to the AV node. This complication is usually transient though.

Lown–Ganong–Levine syndrome
This is characterized by a short PR interval with normal QRS complexes (that is, no delta wave) and paroxysmal AV re-entry tachycardias. Historically, the accessory pathway (Mahaim pathway) is said to connect the AV node to the ventricles or bundle branches but this remains controversial and has not been demonstrated histologically or electrophysiologically.

CARDIOLOGY

1.9

a) Atrial flutter with 2:1 block.

b) The causes of atrial flutter, atrial fibrillation (AF) and atrial tachycardia are the same and are listed in Box 1.1. The commonest causes are probably hypertension, ischaemic heart disease and mitral regurgitation, although in a publican one must clearly consider alcohol, and thyrotoxicosis should always be excluded.

Box 1.1 Causes of atrial fibrillation/atrial flutter

1. Increased atrial pressure
    Hypertension
    Pulmonary embolus
    ASD
    Mitral stenosis/regurgitation
    Congestive cardiac failure
    HOCM
2. Ischaemic heart disease
3. Thyrotoxicosis
4. Alcohol
5. Sino-atrial disease (sick sinus syndrome)
6. Pneumonia
7. Pericarditis/myocarditis
8. Infiltration (e.g. tumour, amyloid)
9. Constrictive pericarditis
10. WPW syndrome
11. Idiopathic (lone AF)

c) In this case the atrial flutter is of recent onset (< 48 h) therefore the treatment of choice is anti-coagulation with intravenous heparin followed by elective synchronized DC cardioversion (see below).

Atrial flutter produces a characteristic 'saw tooth' pattern on the ECG (flutter waves) with an atrial rate of about 300/min.

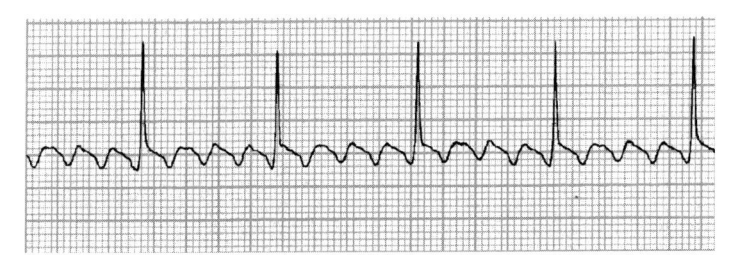

Fig. 1.21 Atrial flutter with 4:1 block

Atrial flutter is usually associated with some degree of AV block so that the ventricular rate is somewhat less than 300/min. When 2:1 block is present (as with the patient in this question) a regular ventricular response rate of about 150/min is produced so that every second flutter wave is masked by a QRS complex thus obscuring the diagnosis. Atrial flutter with 2:1 block is relatively common and it is said that a regular tachycardia of 150/min with narrow QRS complexes should be regarded as atrial flutter with 2:1 block until proven otherwise.

1.10

a) Digoxin.

b) Digoxin toxicity.

An elderly patient who announces that she is on 'heart pills' is most likely to be receiving treatment for angina, heart failure or atrial fibrillation (atrial fibrillation is found in 5–10% of elderly patients). The ECG shows ventricular bigeminy (a ventricular ectopic beat following each sinus beat). The patient also complains of nausea. Ventricular premature beats are the most common rhythm disturbance seen with digoxin toxicity and bigeminy are particularly common in this context. In addition, gastrointestinal symptoms occur frequently in digoxin toxicity. Thus digoxin treatment complicated by digoxin toxicity must feature very high up the list of differential diagnoses.

In most cases of digoxin toxicity discontinuation of digoxin and correction of any hypokalaemia are all that is required although serious ventricular tachyarrhythmias should be treated with intravenous anti-arrhythmic drugs. Phenytoin is useful in this situation (this is about the only situation where phenytoin is still used as an anti-arrhythmic drug) although lignocaine or beta-blockers are alternatives. Haemodynamically unstable tachyarrhythmias should be treated with synchronized DC cardioversion. In the presence of potentially life-threatening arrhythmias Digibind will also be required. Digibind consists of Fab antibody fragments (that is, antibodies that lack the Fc portion and therefore cannot bind complement) that bind specifically to digoxin. Dialysis is of no use in digoxin toxicity owing to the high tissue binding of digoxin.

CARDIOLOGY A

1.11

a) Dextrocardia.

b) Kartagener syndrome.

c) Situs inversus.

The ECG shows gradual reduction in QRS size from V1 to V6, a negative P wave in lead I and a positive P wave in lead aVR. These features are characteristic of dextrocardia. Dextrocardia may be an isolated finding or may occur as part of 'situs inversus' where all of the organs are 'transposed'. The triad of situs inversus, basal bronchiectasis and sinusitis is known as Kartagener syndrome. Bronchiectasis and sinusitis occur in Kartagener syndrome as a result of impaired mucus clearance resulting from abnormal, immotile cilia. The presence of immotile cilia also results in infertility.

1.12

a) The ECG shows right atrial hypertrophy (indicated by the presence of tall peaked P waves) and right ventricular hypertrophy with strain (right ventricular hypertrophy is indicated by the presence of a dominant R wave in V1, a dominant S wave in V6, and right axis deviation of +110 degrees or more. Strain is indicated by ST depression across the right-sided chest leads, V1 to V3 and in the inferior leads, II, III and aVF). Right bundle branch block is also present and frequently accompanies right ventricular hypertrophy (the presence of LBBB would suggest an ostium primum ASD as the underlying cause).

Box 1.2   Causes of a dominant R wave in lead V1
1. Right bundle branch block
2. Right ventricular hypertrophy
3. True posterior MI
4. Wolff–Parkinson–White syndrome type A
5. Dextrocardia
6. Duchenne muscular dystrophy

b) In a person of this age pulmonary hypertension (defined as a systolic pulmonary arterial pressure > 30 mm Hg or a mean arterial pressure > 20 mm Hg) is the most likely cause of hypertrophy of the right-sided chambers. Pulmonary stenosis would need to be considered in a child.

c) The causes of pulmonary hypertension are shown in Box 1.3. In a previously healthy person, however, the most likely causes are recurrent pulmonary emboli, chronic left to right shunting of blood (for example ASD, VSD or PDA) or primary pulmonary hypertension. One must also consider amphetamine-type 'slimming tablets' as a cause, particularly in a woman of this age.

Box 1.3 Causes of pulmonary hypertension

1. Primary pulmonary hypertension (i.e. idiopathic)
2. Secondary causes
   a) Multiple pulmonary emboli
      Thromboembolism
      Amniotic fluid embolism
      Foreign body embolism (i.v. drug abusers)
      Tumour embolism
   b) Chronic left to right shunting of blood (ASD, VSD, PDA)
   c) Chronic hypoxia
      Chronic lung disease
         Restrictive e.g. fibrosis
         Obstructive e.g. chronic bronchitis/emphysema
      Skeletal deformity of chest wall (restrictive defect)
      Weakness of respiratory muscles (restrictive defect)
      Living at high altitude
   d) Pulmonary venous congestion (mitral stenosis, left atrial myxoma)
   e) Autoimmune diseases
      Collagen vascular diseases (SLE, PAN, systemic sclerosis, dermatomyositis, polymyositis)
      Rheumatoid arthritis and juvenile rheumatoid arthritis
      Goodpasture syndrome
      Sarcoidosis
      Fibrosing alveolitis
   f) Sickle cell disease
   g) Parasitic lung disease
      Schistosomiasis (*mansoni* mainly but *japonicum* also)
      Filariasis
   h) Cirrhosis/portal hypertension (mechanism unknown)
   i) Drugs (e.g. certain types of amphetamine-type slimming pills)

CARDIOLOGY

1.13

a) Inferolateral myocardial infarction.

The ECG shows Q waves, ST segment elevation and T wave inversion in the inferior leads (II, III and aVF) and the lateral chest leads (V4 to V6). The MI is probably of a few hours' duration since Q waves and T wave inversion have already occurred.

b) Complete heart block.

The P waves are completely dissociated from the QRS complexes indicating complete heart block. This is a common complication of inferior MI.

1.14

a) The ECG shows broad QRS complexes with tented T waves. This is characteristic of hyperkalaemia.

b) Hyperkalaemia resulting from worsening renal function.

Hyperkalaemia
Increasing hyperkalaemia causes tall, tented T waves followed by reduced P waves with widened QRS complexes. In severe hyperkalaemia the QRS complex may be widened to such a degree that a 'sine wave' pattern is produced. This is usually followed by cardiac arrest which may be of the asystole or electromechanical dissociation variety.

Hypokalaemia
The ECG changes that occur in hypokalaemia are small or inverted P waves, prominent U wave, prolonged PR interval and ST depression. Unlike hyperkalaemia the ECG changes in hypokalaemia correlate poorly with the development of serious dysrhythmias.

1.15

a) Ventricular tachycardia (VT).

The ECG shows a broad complex tachycardia. These can be caused by VT or supraventricular tachycardia (SVT) with aberrant conduction (rate related bundle branch block). However, the 7th QRS complex has a different morphology from the other QRS complexes. This is a 'capture beat' and in the presence of a broad complex tachycardia it is diagnostic of VT. It occurs when the timing of an atrial impulse is such that it can activate the ventricles before the next discharge from the ventricular focus, resulting in a normal QRS complex.

Fusion beats are a similar phenomenon and are also diagnostic of VT. They occur when an atrial beat is transmitted to the ventricles just after the ventricular focus has discharged resulting in a QRS complex that has the appearance of a fusion between a normal QRS complex and a ventricular ectopic beat. Other features that can be used to distinguish whether a broad complex tachycardia is the result of VT or SVT with aberrant conduction are shown in Box 1.4.

Box 1.4 ECG features suggestive of SVT versus VT in the presence of a broad complex tachycardia

Supraventricular tachycardia	Ventricular tachycardia
1. P waves associated with QRS complexes	1. Visible P–QRS dissociation
2. Classical RBBB morphology	2. LBBB morphology
3. Same QRS morphology as in sinus rhythm	3. Fusion/capture beats
4. QRS duration < 0.14 s	4. QRS duration > 0.14 s
5. Normal axis	5. Marked LAD/RAD
	6. Concordant pattern in chest leads (complexes all positive or all negative)

1.16

a) Trifascicular heart block.

b) Insertion of a dual chamber cardiac pacemaker.

Trifascicular block is the combination of prolonged PR interval (first-degree heart block), right bundle branch block and left anterior hemiblock (block of the anterior fascicle of the left Purkinje bundle, which is indicated by left axis deviation). If it is accompanied by syncope and/or intermittent complete heart block there is an increased risk of sudden death and cardiac pacing is indicated. A dual chamber pacemaker is preferred for the pacing of patients with normal atrial contraction (in other words, not in AF) to avoid development of 'pacemaker syndrome'. This occurs when loss of AV synchrony produced by failing to pace both the atrium and the ventricles results in atrial contraction against closed mitral and tricuspid valves. The atrial pressure rises thereby impeding venous return so that during the next diastole the ventricles are not adequately filled. Cardiac output is compromised resulting in hypotension ± syncope or near-syncope. Retrograde (ventriculoatrial) conduction compounds this problem.

1.17

a) Prolongation of the QT interval.
b) Torsade de pointes ventricular tachycardia.
c) Amiodarone therapy for maintenance of sinus rhythm.

The QT interval is measured from the beginning of the QRS complex to the end of the T wave (see Fig. 1.20). It is normally less than about 0.40 s but since the QT interval varies inversely with heart rate a corrected value (QT_c) is conventionally calculated (by dividing by the square root of the R–R interval; see Table 1.2) to adjust for this effect. The normal value for the QT_c is < 0.42 s. In this patient the QT is approximately 0.64 s and the R–R interval is approximately 0.94 s. Therefore the $QT_c = 0.64 / \sqrt{0.94} = 0.66$ s. Prolongation of the QT interval predisposes to ventricular arrhythmias, particularly torsade de pointes ventricular tachycardia.

Some causes of prolonged QT are shown in Box 1.5.

Box 1.5 Causes of prolonged QT interval

1. Electrolyte disturbances
    Hypokalaemia
    Hypocalcaemia
    Hypomagnesaemia

2. Drugs
    Class IA anti-arrhythmics (quinidine, disopyramide, procainamide)
    Class III anti-arrhythmics (amiodarone, sotalol)
    Psychotropics (phenothiazines, tri- and tetracyclic anti-depressants)

3. Central nevous system diseases
    Subarachnoid haemorrhage
    Cryptococcal meningitis

4. Myocardial ischaemia
5. Hypothermia

6. Congenital
    Romano–Ward syndrome (autosomal dominant)
    Jervel–Lange–Nielson syndrome (associated with sensorineural deafness, autosomal recessive)

ECHOCARDIOGRAPHY

Any echocardiograms encountered in the MRCP exam will almost certainly be either the parasternal long axis or apical four-chamber views.

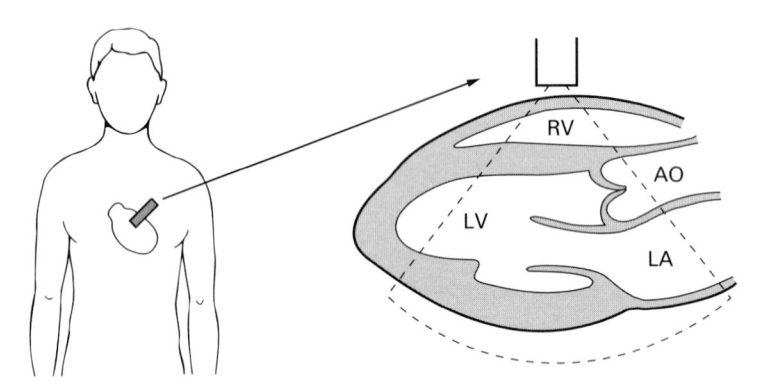

Fig. 1.22 Schematic diagram of parasternal long axis image plane

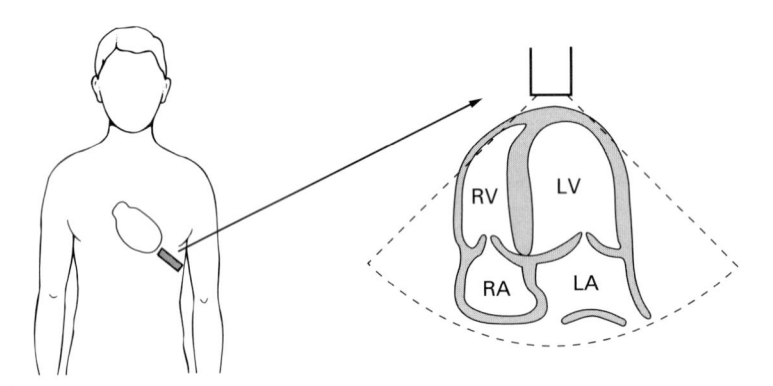

Fig. 1.23 Schematic diagram of apical four-chamber image plane

The echo machine usually has four modes, but only the M-mode or 2D imaging modes are likely to be examined:

M-mode

M-mode (time motion scanning) analyses the signal from a single scan line and displays the data as a graph of echo signal depths against time. M-mode allows wall and/or valve cusp motion to be examined at a particular point along the scanning plane, for example sampling across the mitral valve in the parasternal long axis plane as in Fig. 1.24.

CARDIOLOGY

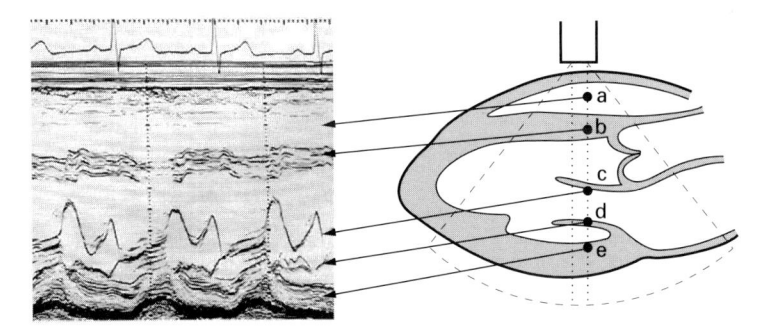

Fig. 1.24 M-mode echocardiogram in the parasternal long axis plane, sampling at the point of the mitral valve leaflets. a = right ventricle; b = interventricular septum; c = anterior mitral valve leaflet; d = posterior mitral valve leaflet; e = posterior wall of left ventricle

A number of cardiac conditions can be diagnosed from the abnormal patterns of mitral valve motion that they produce (Fig. 1.25).

The dimensions of the ventricles are measured at a point just beyond the tips of the mitral valve leaflets (at the level of the chordae tendinae) and the dimensions of the aortic root and LA are measured at the level of the aortic valve. These are shown schematically in Figs 1.26 and 1.27, below. Although the echocardiograph calculates these dimensions automatically after the operator has selected the points at which to measure, the M-mode trace has vertical marks placed 1 cm apart, which allows one to measure the chamber sizes directly during the exam. Ventricular measurements are usually taken at both end diastole (meaning at the point of the Q wave on the ECG trace) and end systole (for ventricular measurements this is taken as the most posterior septal motion point or the most anterior motion point of the LVPW). The aortic root diameter is measured at end diastole (as defined by the ECG) whereas the left atrial dimension is measured at end systole (for measurement of the LA dimension end systole is defined by closure of the aortic valve and the maximum atrial dimension that occurs around this point is measured).

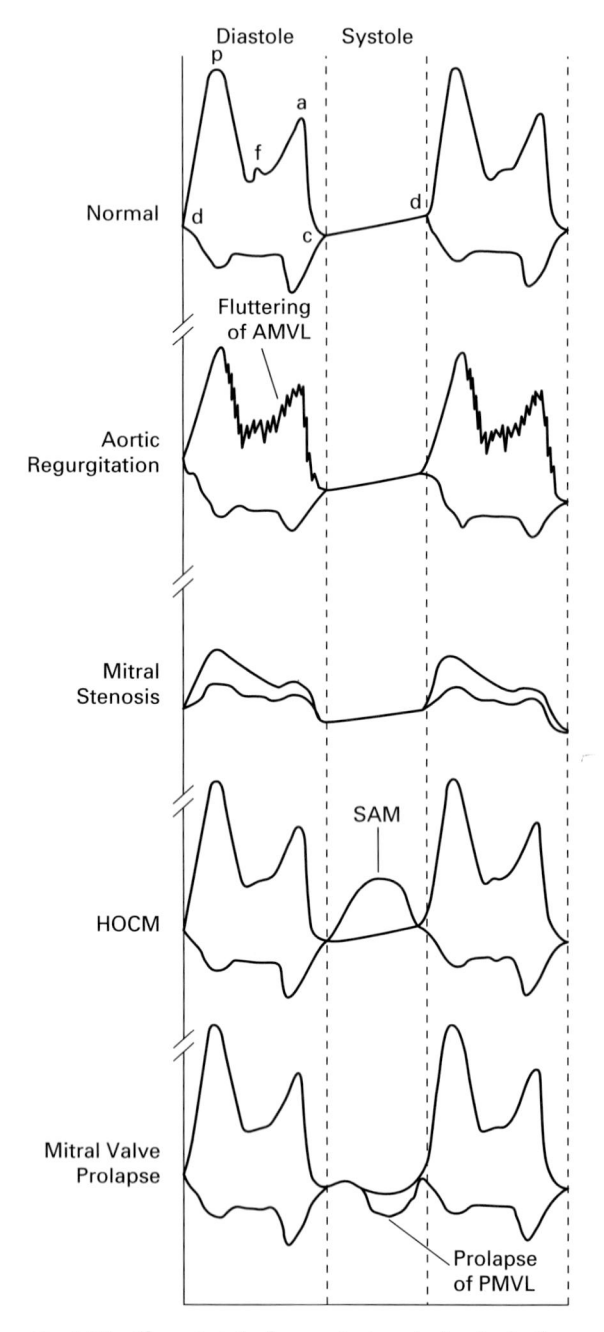

Fig. 1.25 Characteristic changes in the mitral valve leaflet waveform that are seen with various cardiac abnormalities. SAM = systolic anterior motion

CARDIOLOGY

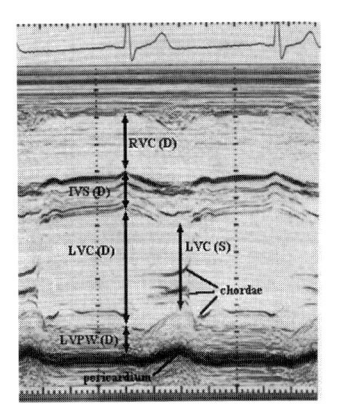

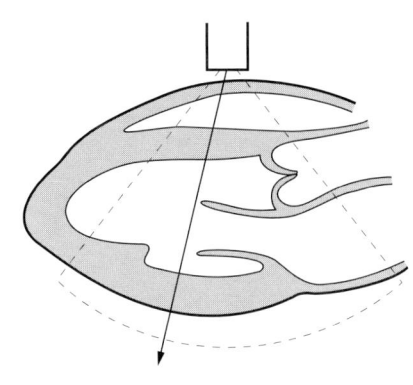

Fig. 1.26 M-mode recording in the parasternal long axis plane taken at a point just beyond the tips of the mitral valve leaflets, at the level of the chordae tendinae. RVC (D) = right ventricular cavity dimension at end diastole; IVS (D) = interventricular septum thickness at end diastole; LVC (D) = left ventricular cavity dimension at end diastole; LVPW (D) = left ventricular posterior wall thickness at end diastole; LVC (S) = left ventricular cavity dimension at end systole

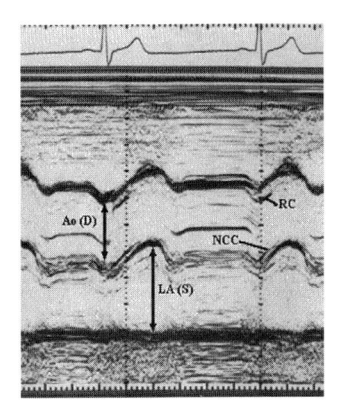

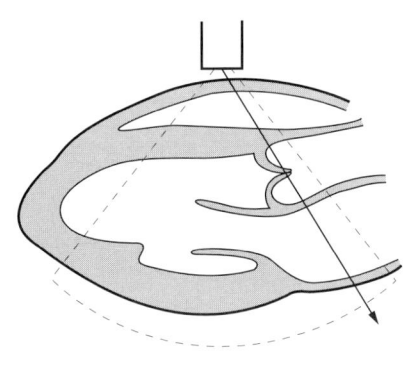

Fig. 1.27 M-mode recording taken in the parasternal long axis plane at the level of the aortic root: Ao (D) = aortic root dimension at end diastole; LA (S) = left atrial cavity dimension at end systole; RC = right cusp of aortic valve; NCC = non-coronary cusp of aortic valve

Table 1.3 Approximate normal values of M-mode echocardiographic measurements (adults)*

	Size (cm)
RVC (D)	0.7–2.6
IVS (D)	0.6–1.1
LVC (D)	3.5–5.6
LVC (S)	2.0–3.7
LVPW (D)	0.6–1.2
Ao (D)	2.0–3.7
LA (S)	1.9–4.0

*The exact range of normal values varies depending upon the echo machine that is used and the population studied; therefore only approximate values can be given here

1.18

a) This is an M-mode echocardiogram taken at the level of the mitral valve leaflets in the parasternal long axis plane. It shows asymmetric septal hypertrophy and systolic anterior motion (SAM) of the anterior mitral valve leaflet.

b) Hypertrophic obstructive cardiomyopathy (HOCM).

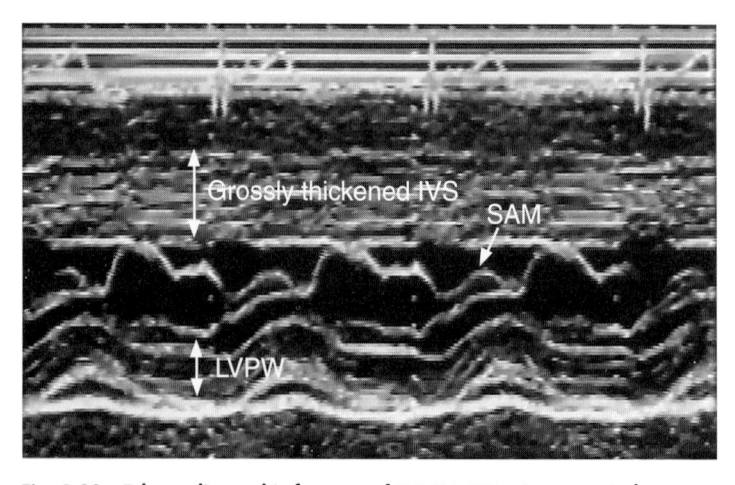

Fig. 1.28 Echocardiographic features of HOCM: IVS = interventricular septum; LVPW = left ventricular posterior wall; SAM = systolic anterior movement of anterior mitral valve leaflet

CARDIOLOGY

Hypertrophic cardiomyopathy

Hypertrophic cardiomyopathy (HCM) is caused by a single gene defect. In 50% of cases it is inherited as an autosomal dominant trait with a high degree of penetrance; the remainder of cases are sporadic. Mutations have been identified in the β-myosin heavy chain, tropomyosin and troponin T genes. HCM is characterized by left and/or right ventricular hypertrophy in the absence of an identifiable cause. It most frequently affects the interventricular septum (asymmetric septal hypertrophy) and a ratio of septal thickness:left ventricular posterior wall thickness of > 1.5, with an absolute septal thickness > 1.4 cm, is highly suggestive of this condition. Hypertrophic obstructive cardiomyopathy (HOCM) is a variant of HCM. In addition to the other features of HCM, HOCM is characterized by anterior movement of the anterior mitral valve leaflet during systole (systolic anterior motion). As a result the anterior mitral valve leaflet becomes opposed to the interventricular septum and, since the grossly thickened septum protrudes into the LV outflow tract, LV outflow obstruction occurs in late systole.

Most patients with HCM are asymptomatic and it therefore often presents with sudden death caused by arrhythmia. The most common symptoms are:

- *Exertional dyspnoea* caused by a number of factors including impaired LV filling, elevation of LA and pulmonary venous pressures, and, later in the course of the disease, heart failure.
- *Chest pain* which may be overt angina secondary to the increased oxygen demands of the hypertrophied myocardium (± coronary artery disease), or atypical chest pain of unknown aetiology.
- *Palpitations* secondary to supraventricular and ventricular arrhythmias.
- *Syncope (especially exertional)* may be the result of inadequate cardiac output on exertion or cardiac arrhythmias.

1.19

a) This is an M-mode echocardiogram taken at the level of the mitral valve in the parasternal long axis plane. It shows thickened mitral valve leaflets (indicated by echo reduplication), loss of the classic 'M' shape of the anterior mitral valve leaflet, and the posterior mitral valve leaflet moving anteriorly rather than posteriorly during diastole.

b) The above changes are indicative of mitral stenosis.

This patient is also in AF, as indicated by both the ECG trace at the top of the image and the beat to beat variation in the duration of diastole (the duration of mitral valve cusp separation varies from beat to beat). Patients with clinically significant mitral stenosis are often in AF and, for the purposes of the MRCP exam, the presence of AF on the echo trace may give a clue as to the diagnosis.

c) This patient has had a stroke caused by systemic embolization of atrial thrombus resulting from atrial fibrillation.

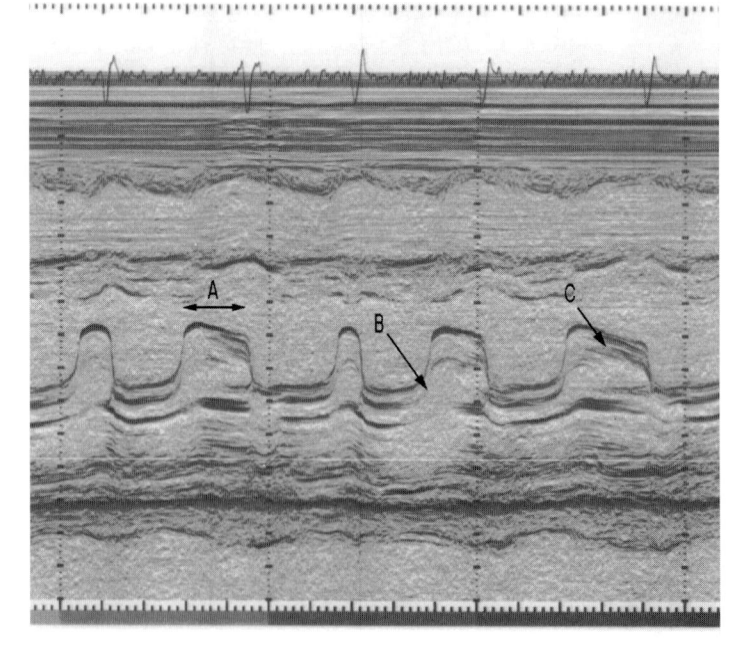

Fig. 1.29 M-mode trace at the level of the mitral valve, in the parasternal long axis plane, showing the typical changes of mitral stenosis: A = loss of 'M' and 'W' shaped waveforms of the anterior and posterior leaflets; B = anterior movement of posterior leaflet during diastole; C = echo reduplication around mitral valve leaflets

Although the characteristic changes of mitral stenosis are often best seen on the M-mode trace, the severity of stenosis is assessed on 2D echo by measuring the area of the mitral valve orifice on the parasternal short axis view. In normal adults the mitral valve orifice area is 3–5 cm^2. Moderate stenosis is said to be present when the valve area is reduced to 1–1.5 cm^2 and severe stenosis is defined by a valve area < 1 cm^2.

1.20

a) The echocardiogram shows the presence of a pericardial effusion.

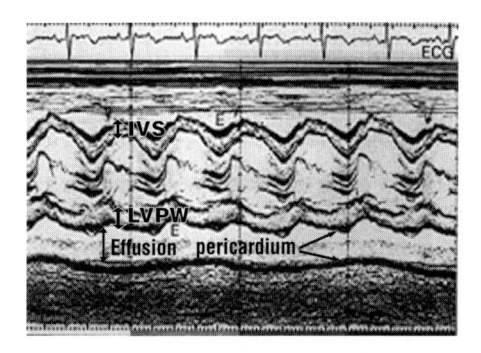

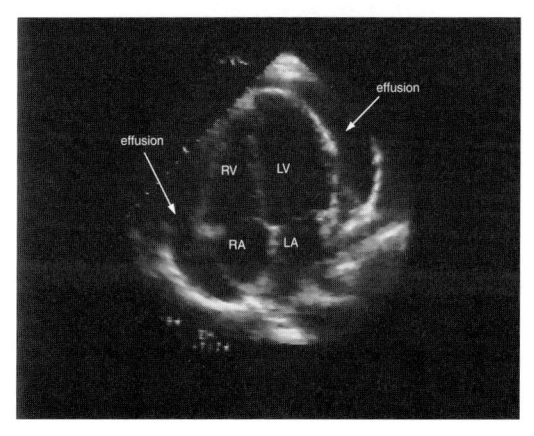

Fig. 1.30 and 1.31 M-mode and 2D echocardiograms in the parasternal long axis plane showing the presence of a pericardial effusion: IVS = interventricular septum; LVPW = left ventricular posterior wall

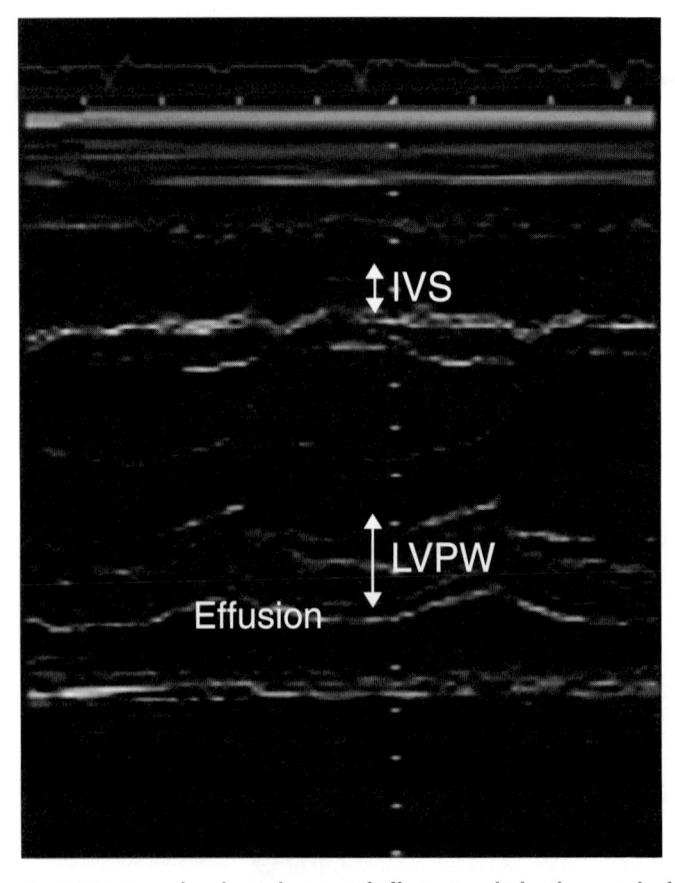

Fig. 1.32 M-mode echocardiogram of effusion in which echos are displayed in white on a black background and the effusion therefore appears as a black echo-free space (parasternal long axis)

A pericardial effusion is an abnormal collection of fluid within the pericardial space (i.e. > 50 ml fluid) and appears as an 'echo-free' zone between the ventricular wall and the pericardium. Since fluid tends to gravitate posteriorly, effusions are best seen on the parasternal long axis view behind the left ventricular wall. By convention tissue echoes are usually (but not always: see Q 1.18 and Q 1.21, and Fig. 1.32) displayed in black on a white background in M-mode and in white on a black background during 2D echo. Thus, in M-mode the effusion appears as a white space between the signal from the

LPVW and that from the pericardium, whereas in 2D echo the effusion appears as a black space. Diastolic collapse of the RA and particularly the RV may also be seen on the 2D echo and if present are indicative of cardiac tamponade.

b) The most likely cause in this case is direct infiltration of the pericardium as a result of extension of the patient's small cell carcinoma of the bronchus, although metastatic spread could also be a cause.

c) An elevated JVP with Kussmaul's sign are characteristic of a pericardial effusion. Kussmaul's sign consists of a paradoxical rise in the JVP during inspiration – normally the JVP should fall during inspiration as negative intrathoracic pressure 'sucks' blood from the great veins into the chest. Kussmaul's sign is not specific for pericardial effusion and may also occur with constrictive pericarditis and cardiogenic shock as a result of right ventricular infarct.

Box 1.6 Causes of pericarditis and pericardial effusion

1. Viral myocarditis (mainly Coxsackie A and B; others include HIV, mumps, VZV, influenza and EBV)
2. **T**rauma and **TB**
3. **U**raemia
4. **M**yocardial infarct and **M**edications e.g. procainamide, hydralazine
5. **O**ther infections (bacterial, fungal, TB)
6. **R**heumatoid arthritis and other autoimmune disorders; **R**adiation

   The mnemonic **TUMOR** is a reminder that metastatic and infiltrative cancer are also frequent causes. Cardiac metastases may be seen with bronchogenic carcinoma, breast carcinoma, leukaemia, lymphoma and malignant melanoma.

7. Dressler syndrome (post myocardial infarction syndrome)
8. Hypothyroidism

1.21

a) Left atrial myxoma.

b) Serial blood cultures.

The symptoms, signs and haematological results are compatible with a diagnosis of either mitral stenosis complicated by infective endocarditis, or a left atrial myxoma. Faced with these clinical findings appropriate investigations should include transoesophageal echocardiography and serial blood cultures to exclude endocarditis. In this case the echocardiogram demonstrates the classical M-mode characteristics of left atrial myxoma (below) together with a filling defect in the left atrium, seen on the 2D echo. Blood cultures are still indicated however since myxomata can be the focus of endocarditis.

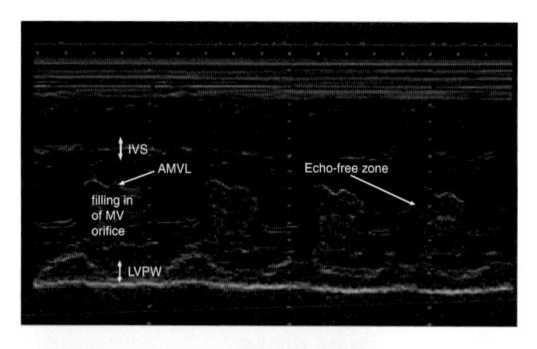

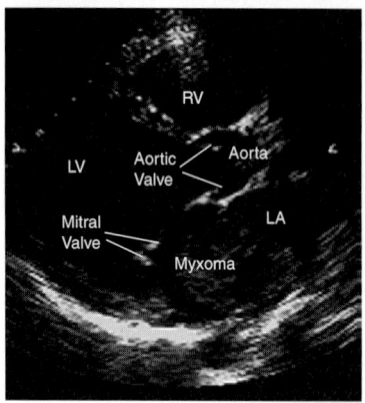

Fig. 1.33 and 1.34 M-mode and 2D echocardiograms in the parasternal long axis planes showing the presence of a left atrial myxoma: IVS = interventricular septum; LVPW = left ventricular posterior wall; AMVL = anterior mitral valve leaflet

CARDIOLOGY

Myxomata are the commonest primary tumours of the heart (in adults) and although they can occur in any of the cardiac chambers 75% arise in the left atrium (LA). They tend to prolapse into the mitral valve (MV) orifice during diastole producing a high pitched early diastolic sound (a 'tumour plop') and obstruction to MV blood flow that can be heard on auscultation as a mid-diastolic murmur. The haemodynamic consequences of obstruction to MV blood flow mean that LA myxomata often present with symptoms similar to those of mitral stenosis. This, together with the mid-diastolic murmur and the fact that a tumour plop sounds similar to an opening snap, means that the clinical picture of LA myxoma can almost exactly mimic that of mitral stenosis. Myxomata can also present with systemic embolization, sudden death, syncope or constitutional symptoms such as malaise, fever (myxoma is a cause of PUO), weight loss and an elevated ESR. Haemolysis may also occur.

The diagnosis of LA myxoma is made at echocardiography when it can best be seen on the 2D echo as a highly mobile filling defect within the LA. On the M-mode scan the myxoma is seen as a dense mass of echoes between the MV leaflets, causing 'filling in' of the mitral valve orifice during diastole. There is a slight delay (seen as an echo-free zone) between the opening of the MV leaflets and the appearance of the tumour echoes. This corresponds to the time taken for the tumour to prolapse from the LA into the MV orifice and, if presented with only the M-mode trace in the exam, this feature can be used to distinguish LA myxoma from mitral stenosis – echo reduplication in mitral stenosis may also produce the appearance of filling in of the MV orifice.

1.22

a) Mural thrombus in the left ventricle.

b) Anti-coagulation with intravenous heparin followed by oral warfarin for 3–6 months.

Intracardiac thrombi are best detected on 2D echo where they are seen as a filling defect, in close proximity to the wall, within a cardiac chamber. On transthoracic echo they are most commonly seen in the LV in association with a wall motion abnormality (usually following an anterior MI) and are usually situated at the ventricular apex where stasis of blood is most likely to occur. Thrombus formation may also occur in the left or right atrial appendage, particularly in association with AF. However, this part of the atrium is not well visualized on transthoracic echo and transoesophageal echo is therefore required to exclude the presence of thrombus at this site.

LV mural thrombus occurs in 20–40% of patients with anterior myocardial infarction and thrombotic risk is directly related to infarct size. Embolization may result in stroke, critical limb ischaemia, and renal, splenic or mesenteric infarction, and usually occurs within the first 10 days of MI. Pedunculated thrombi are the most likely to embolize. Treatment is with anti-coagulation for 3–6 months.

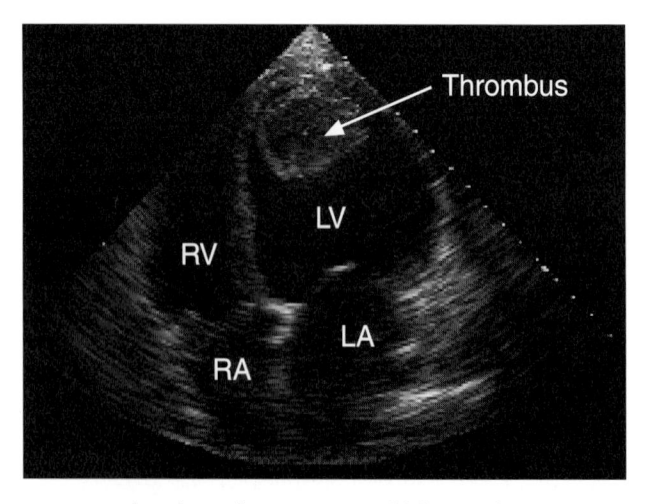

Fig. 1.35 Thrombus adherent to apex of left ventricle

CARDIOLOGY

RADIONUCLIDE IMAGING

Radionuclide imaging is a non-invasive imaging technique during which a radiolabelled substance is injected into a peripheral blood vessel and a gamma camera is used to detect radioactivity transmitted back from the region of the heart. This radioactive 'signal' is then used to construct an image of the heart. There are a number of different radionuclide imaging techniques but these can be broadly divided into two categories:

1. Myocardial perfusion scanning
2. Functional imaging.

For the purpose of the MRCP written exam, perfusion imaging is the only technique that is likely to be examined.

MYOCARDIAL PERFUSION SCANNING
Thallium scan

This imaging modality is used to diagnose myocardial ischaemia and utilizes a radiolabelled tracer that is taken up by cardiac myocytes. Distribution of the tracer is dependent upon regional myocardial blood flow and regions of myocardial ischaemia will therefore show up as 'cold' spots on the image. Exercise in the form of a standard exercise tolerance test is usually used to induce ischaemia although pharmacologically induced stress, using vasodilator agents such as dipyridamole or adenosine, is an alternative for patients who are unable to perform an exercise test. Images are taken in several planes allowing most regions of the left ventricular myocardium to be visualized. However, since the atria and right ventricle are thin walled they don't usually take up enough tracer to show up on the scan.

The most widely used tracer is thallium-201 and consequently the term 'thallium scan' has become synonymous with 'myocardial perfusion scan'. Thallium-201 is only taken up by viable myocytes which means that areas of ischaemia and areas of dead myocardium (that is, old infarcts) will both show up as cold spots. In order to differentiate between the two it is necessary to repeat the thallium scan after a few hours of rest (usually about 4 h after the exercise test). During this rest period redistribution of the tracer occurs as blood flow returns to the ischaemic myocardium.

Thus cold spots caused by ischaemia will not show up on the second scan (they are said to be reversible) whereas cold spots caused by dead myocardium will persist. Technetium-99 m labelled compounds are often used as an alternative to thallium-201.

Single photon emission computerized tomography (SPECT)

For the purposes of MRCP data interpretation, this differs from planar thallium-201 (or technetium-99) scanning only in the fact that it allows tomographic (cross-sectional) images of the heart to be obtained. This is achieved by rotating the gamma camera through 180° around the patient, from the right anterior oblique 30° to left posterior oblique 30°, acquiring information at 6° intervals. Computerized image reconstruction can generate slices at approximately 1 cm intervals and both short- and long-axis views can be evaluated. The exercise and resting images are interpreted in the same way as a standard perfusion scan.

Infarct-avid imaging (hotspot scanning)

This uses a radiolabelled substance that is selectively taken up by acutely injured myocytes and thus outlines acute myocardial infarction as a 'hotspot'. A number of different tracers can be used for this purpose. Since perfusion scanning shows up abnormalities as cold spots, the presence of a hotspot on a cardiac radionuclide image in the MRCP should alert you to the fact that the question relates to infarct-avid imaging rather than perfusion imaging. The presence of the hotspot is itself diagnostic and gives you the answer without much in the way of interpretation being necessary.

1.23

a) Myocardial infarction.

b) 300 mg soluble aspirin.

Although the ECG is normal, the thallium (SPECT) scan clearly shows a perfusion defect (arrowed in Fig. 1.37). This defect is not reversible after a few hours' rest indicating that it is caused by dead myocardium (that is, MI) rather than a perfusion defect. All patients with ischaemic heart disease should receive aspirin unless contraindicated. In the presence of acute ischaemia the initial dose should be 300 mg in order to achieve immediate platelet inhibition. Subsequent doses can be 75 mg per day.

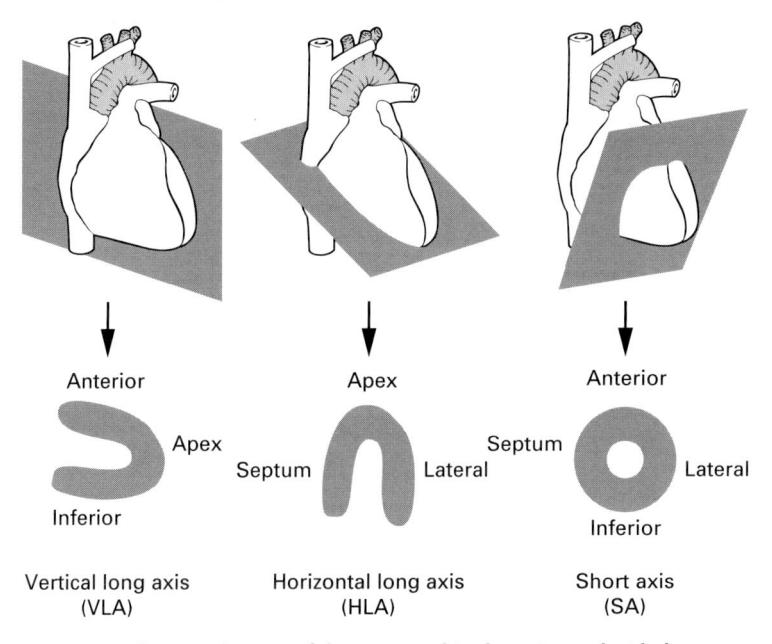

Fig. 1.36 Schematic diagram of the tomographic planes imaged with the thallium scan (Based on D. J. Pennell and E. Prvulovich, Nuclear Cardiology, British Nuclear Medicine Society 1995, p. 58, with permission)

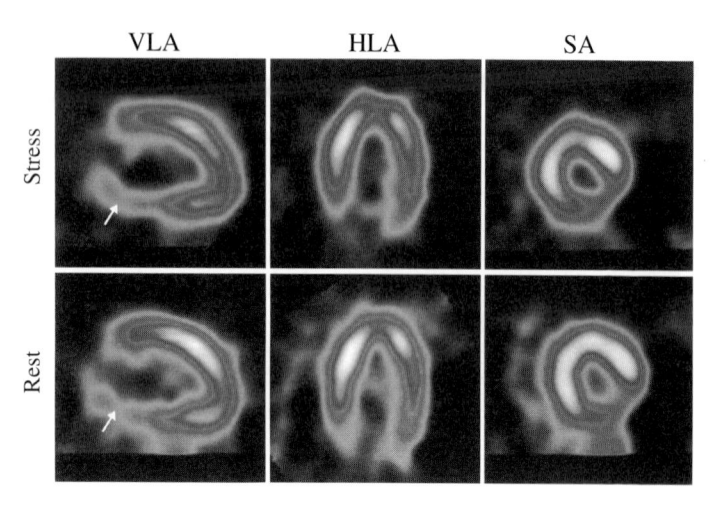

Fig. 1.37 Thallium scan showing an inferior MI: there is a perfusion defect (arrowed) on exercise in the territory of the right coronary artery that is not reversed following a few hours' rest (From D. J. Pennell and E. Prvulovich: Nuclear Cardiology, British Nuclear Medicine Society 1995, p. 92, with permission)

The changes that would be seen on the thallium scan of a patient with angina alone are shown in Fig. 1.38.

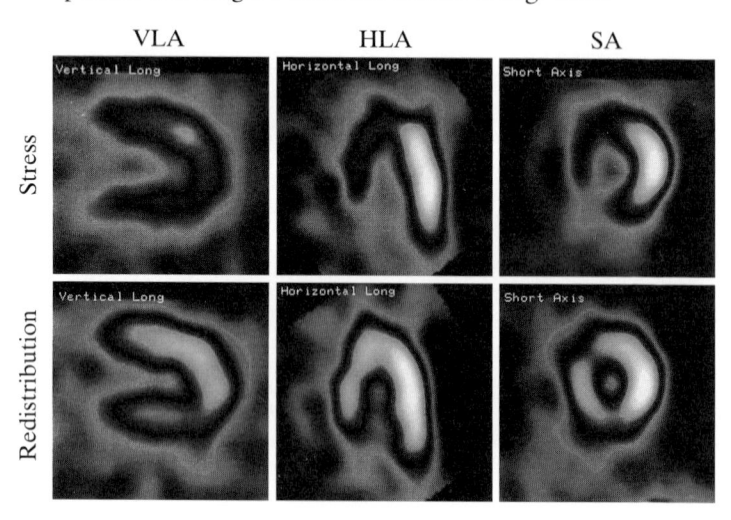

Fig. 1.38 Thallium scan showing multi-vessel disease in a patient with angina: there is reduced tracer uptake in the anterior wall, septum, inferior wall and apex on exercise that is reversed in the redistribution images (Image provided by Dr E. Prvulovich, Consultant Physician in Nuclear Medicine, University College London Medical School)

2 ENDOCRINOLOGY

PITUITARY-ADRENAL AXIS

2.1

a) Cushing syndrome.

Hypokalaemic alkalosis is suggestive of excess mineralocorticoid activity; this does not however explain the high blood glucose result. Glucocorticoids also have mineralocorticoid activity and this becomes particularly apparent when they are produced in excess, that is, in Cushing syndrome. Excess glucocorticoid levels can also produce glucose intolerance or diabetes. (Hyperventilation can also produce alkalosis and would also account for this patient's shortness of breath. However, hyperventilation is unlikely to be sustained for long enough to produce this degree of hypokalaemia.)

b) Ectopic ACTH production from oat cell carcinoma of the bronchus.

Very low potassium levels, as seen in this case, characteristically occur in Cushing syndrome that is caused by ectopic ACTH production. Ectopic ACTH is most commonly the result of an oat cell carcinoma of the bronchus and this patient's shortness of breath could be indicative of an underlying bronchial tumour.

c) A dexamethasone suppression test (to confirm the diagnosis of Cushing syndrome), 9 a.m. and midnight plasma ACTH (and cortisol) to determine whether the Cushing has an ACTH-dependent cause, and a CXR are all indicated. Subsequent tests might include a high-dose dexamethasone suppression test, CT/MRI of the pituitary fossa and selective venous sampling from the inferior petrosal sinus. 24 h urinary-free cortisol could also be used to confirm the diagnosis of Cushing but this is less sensitive than a dexamethasone suppression test.

d) The muscular weakness could be secondary to proximal myopathy (which is a feature of Cushing syndrome), hypokalaemia, spinal cord compression from bony metastases or an osteopathic fracture (osteoporosis commonly occurs in Cushing), or polymyositis (which may be associated with malignancy).

ENDOCRINOLOGY

Table 2.1 Causes of Cushing syndrome

ACTH-dependent
Excess ACTH secretion → adrenal hyperplasia (diffuse or macronodular) and hypersecretion of cortisol

Pituitary-dependent (Cushing's disease)	• This is the commonest non-iatrogenic cause and accounts for 80% of cases
	• 90% caused by microadenomas; 10% caused by macroadenomas
Ectopic ACTH secretion by tumour	• Oat cell carcinoma of bronchus (50%)
	• Some carcinoid tumours: lung (15%); other (5%)
	• Pancreas
	• Medullary cell carcinoma of thyroid

Non-ACTH-dependent
Excess cortisol → suppression of ACTH secretion
Adrenal causes

Adenoma	• Accounts for 10% of non-iatrogenic Cushing
Carcinoma	• Accounts for 10% of non-iatrogenic Cushing
	• Commonest cause in children
	• Usually secrete other adrenal hormones as well → hirsutism/virilization in women

Iatrogenic
  Glucocorticoid/ACTH administration
Other

Pseudo-Cushing	• Caused by alcoholism or depression
	• Patients with pseudo-Cushing show many of the same biochemical features as true Cushing including loss of circadian rhythm, ↑ urinary-free cortisol and failure to suppress with a 48 h (low-dose) dexamethasone suppression test
	• Insulin stress test may be helpful to distinguish pseudo-Cushing from true Cushing
Rare syndromes	• Carney syndrome
	• McCune–Albright syndrome

INVESTIGATION OF CUSHING SYNDROME

Investigation of Cushing consists of tests to confirm the diagnosis, tests to determine the cause and imaging to localize the cause. Tests to confirm the diagnosis are listed below. The dexamethasone suppression test is the most sensitive indicator and should therefore always be quoted in preference to the other tests in answer to MRCP questions.

- *24h urinary-free cortisol*: This is elevated in Cushing syndrome.
- *9 a.m. and midnight plasma cortisol (and ACTH)*: The normal diurnal variation in cortisol synthesis is lost in Cushing syndrome so the midnight level will be high (9 a.m. cortisol may also be high). ACTH is often measured as well since this will show whether the Cushing is ACTH-dependent or not.
- *Dexamethasone suppression test*: In normal individuals administration of dexamethasone causes suppression of cortisol synthesis by inhibiting ACTH release from the anterior pituitary. An overnight test is performed initially as a screening test. This has a high sensitivity but low specificity (false positive results occur in about 10% of cases); if this is positive it is therefore customary to perform a 48 h dexamethasone test to confirm the results. The high-dose dexamethasone suppression test is used to distinguish between pituitary-dependent and ectopic ACTH production (see below).

Table 2.2 Dexamethasone suppression test

	Positive (normal) test
Overnight test 1 mg dexamethasone taken orally at 22.00 h Plasma cortisol measured at 09.00 h the next day	• Cortisol < 180 nmol/L
48 h test 0.5 mg dexamethasone taken orally, 6 hourly, for 2 days. Plasma cortisol measured at start and at 09.00 h on day 3	• Cortisol < 180 nmol/L on second sample
High-dose test (two methods) a) Same as low-dose test but 2 mg of dexamethasone used	• Cortisol suppressed to less than 50% of initial value
or b) Basal blood sample taken at 08.00 h 8 mg of dexamethasone given at 22.00 h the same day and repeat blood sample taken at 08.00 h the following morning	• Cortisol suppressed to less than 50% of initial value

ENDOCRINOLOGY

- *Insulin stress test*: This is used to differentiate pseudo-Cushing (caused by alcoholism or depression) from true Cushing. In true Cushing there is a flat cortisol response (that is, no rise) to insulin-induced hypoglycaemia whereas in pseudo-Cushing (and normal individuals) the plasma cortisol rises in response to stress. It is important to make sure that adequate hypoglycaemia (< 2.2 mmol/L) has occurred.

Tests to determine the cause of elevated glucocorticoid levels are listed below. ACTH levels and high-dose dexamethasone test are the most discriminatory and should therefore be performed first (in other words, these are the ones that should be quoted first in MRCP exam answers). The other tests are listed mainly so that you will know how to interpret them if they come up in the exam:

- *9 a.m. and midnight ACTH levels*: These are used to discriminate between ACTH-dependent (ACTH levels high; typically very high in ectopic ACTH secretion) and non-ACTH-dependent (ACTH secretion greatly suppressed) Cushing.
- *High-dose dexamethasone suppression test*: This is used to discriminate between pituitary-dependent excess ACTH secretion and excess ACTH caused by secretion from an ectopic source. Pituitary adenomas remain partially responsive to feedback inhibition by cortisol, albeit at a higher level, and ACTH secretion (and hence cortisol secretion) is therefore suppressed during the high-dose test. This is not the case with ectopic ACTH secretion. Adrenal Cushing does not suppress during this test either.
- *Corticotrophin releasing factor (CRF) test*: This is also used to distinguish between pituitary-dependent and ectopic excess ACTH secretion. Administration of CRF produces an increase in ACTH and cortisol levels in pituitary-dependent disease but not in ectopic ACTH secretion or adrenal Cushing. Blood is taken every 15 min following administration of ACTH and a 100% rise in plasma ACTH or a 50% rise in plasma cortisol levels constitutes a positive test.
- *Metyrapone suppression test*: This is another test that can be used to distinguish between pituitary-dependent and ectopic ACTH secretion. The test is now outdated but you

may be asked to interpret the results in the MRCP. Metyrapone inhibits 11 β hydroxylase and thus blocks cortisol synthesis. Since pituitary adenomas remain partially sensitive to feedback inhibition by cortisol, a fall in the plasma cortisol level results in an increase in ACTH release. This is not the case for ectopic ACTH secretion.

Table 2.3 Results of metyrapone suppression test

Cushing's disease	• Metyrapone causes an ↑ in ACTH
Ectopic ACTH secretion	• No ↑ in ACTH with metyrapone

- *Selective venous sampling from inferior petrosal sinus.* The blood from each half of the anterior pituitary drains into the ipsilateral inferior petrosal sinus. Thus ACTH levels in blood sampled from the inferior petrosal sinus will have a higher ACTH concentration than that sampled from a peripheral vein.
- *Selective venous sampling from adrenal veins.* This may be required to demonstrate on which side the adrenal tumour lies if imaging fails to show it.

Imaging consists mainly of CT/MRI of the adrenals and pituitary but should only be interpreted together with the results of the biochemical tests since clinically silent adenomas are often detected. Radioactive isotope scanning using radiolabelled iodocholesterol may be helpful for localizing adrenal tumours that cannot be detected by CT/MRI. Adrenal adenomas take up the tracer with suppression of the surrounding and contralateral adrenal tissue. Carcinomas typically take the tracer up slowly and therefore do not show up, but since the surrounding and contralateral adrenal tissue is suppressed this does not show up either so the scan shows nothing.

ENDOCRINOLOGY

Table 2.4 Interpretation of the tests used for differentiating the cause of Cushing syndrome

	09.00 h plasma ACTH	Dexamethasone suppression test – Overnight	Dexamethasone suppression test – 48 h low dose	Dexamethasone suppression test – 48 h high dose	CRF test	Metyrapone suppression test	Insulin stress test
Pituitary-dependent	↑	–	–	+	+	+	–
Ectopic ACTH	↑↑	–	–	–	–	–	–
Adrenal adenoma	↓	–	–	–	–	–	–
Adrenal carcinoma	↓	–	–	–	–	–	–
Pseudo-Cushing	↓/→	–	+/–	+	•	•	+

+ denotes a positive test; – denotes a negative test. See text for what constitutes + and – in each of these tests.

2.2

a) Pituitary-dependent Cushing syndrome (Cushing's disease), or pseudo-Cushing caused by alcoholism or depression.

b) Insulin stress test with measurement of plasma cortisol and ACTH.

In pituitary-dependent Cushing syndrome excess cortisol secretion is characteristically suppressed by a high-dose dexamethasone suppression test. However pseudo-Cushing can produce both similar dexamethasone suppression test results and a similar clinical picture. An insulin stress test produces a flat cortisol response in Cushing's disease, whereas in pseudo-Cushing there is an increase in cortisol and ACTH in response to stress.

2.3

a) Ectopic ACTH production (for example, from oat cell carcinoma bronchus) or a cortisol-secreting adrenal tumour (adenoma or carcinoma).

b) Plasma ACTH will be high in ectopic ACTH secretion but greatly suppressed in adrenal Cushing.

This patient has an elevated plasma cortisol that is not suppressed during a high-dose dexamethasone suppression test (see Table 2.4). This is characteristic of either ectopic

ACTH production (oat cell carcinoma of the bronchus is the commonest cause) or an adrenal tumour. Although with the majority of pituitary adenomas ACTH secretion is suppressed during a high-dose dexamethasone suppression test, this is not the case in about 10% of cases so additional tests may be necessary to differentiate between pituitary-dependent and ectopic ACTH hypersecretion. These include a CRH test and selective venous sampling from the inferior petrosal sinuses (the metyrapone suppression test is now obsolete). Blurred vision may occur as a result of hyperglycaemia as a result of changes in hydration of the cornea. Headache is a non-specific symptom.

2.4

a) Cushing syndrome caused by an adrenal carcinoma.

Excess cortisol secretion has not been suppressed by a high-dose dexamethasone suppression test (see Table 2.4). This is characteristic of either adrenal Cushing (that is, adrenal adenoma or carcinoma) or ectopic ACTH production. However elevated 17-ketosteroids, which are produced by metabolism of androgens, together with severe hirsutism and male-pattern baldness imply that there is excess androgen production as well as the increased cortisol. This is more characteristic of an adrenal carcinoma.

2.5

a) Primary adrenal failure (Addison's disease).

b) Autoimmune; amyloid; TB; metastases (carcinoma of the bronchus); meningococcal septicaemia (Friderichsen–Waterhouse syndrome).

c) This patient is having an Addisonian crisis. This is a medical emergency and should be treated immediately with intravenous hydrocortisone and colloid (to expand the plasma volume and so elevate the blood pressure). Blood should first be taken for cortisol and ACTH assay if possible. Once she is over the acute crisis hydrocortisone can be switched to dexamethasone (which does not interfere with the assay for cortisol) in order to perform a Synacthen test.

d) Blood should be taken for plasma ACTH and cortisol assay and for glucose measurement. A Synacthen test should also be performed when the patient has recovered from the acute episode.

e) Hyperpigmentation occurs in primary but not secondary adrenal insufficiency.

Low sodium with high potassium is suggestive of failure of mineralocorticoid production, although over-treatment with a thiazide plus a potassium sparing diuretic could produce a similar biochemical picture. Since mineralocorticoid production is unaffected in secondary hypoadrenalism (which is caused by failure of pituitary ACTH secretion), primary adrenal failure (Addison's disease) is the most likely diagnosis.* A degree of renal impairment is also common in Addison's disease, and weight loss, fatigue and abdominal pain are all cardinal symptoms of adrenal failure (primary or secondary).

*Some authorities say that significant hyponatraemia does not occur in pituitary-dependent adrenocortical insufficiency (because of the fact that mineralocorticoid production is independent of ACTH) and that significant hypoglycaemia does not occur in Addison's disease (as a result of continued production of growth hormone by the pituitary). This is controversial and, for the purposes of the MRCP, I would assume that hyponatraemia and hypoglycaemia can occur in both conditions but that hyponatraemia together with hyperkalaemia is more likely to be caused by Addison's, particularly if uraemia is also present.

Table 2.5 Causes of adrenal failure

Primary adrenal failure (Addison's disease)

1. Autoimmune	• Commonest cause (70%)
	• Associated with anti-adrenal antibodies
	• May occur as part of polyglandular deficiency syndrome
2. TB	• Calcified adrenals are characteristic
	• Both the cortex and the medulla are affected
3. Adrenal infarction	
Meningococcal septicaemia	• This is known as Friderichsen–
Complication of venography	Waterhouse syndrome
4. Adrenal infiltration	• Most commonly Ca bronchus
Metastases	
Amyloid	
5. Bilateral adrenalectomy	
6. Adrenal leukodystrophy	• Rare

Secondary adrenal failure

1. Pituitary or hypothalamic disease	• For example: pituitary tumours; post-pituitary surgery or irradiation; postpartum pituitary infarction (Sheehan syndrome); infiltration by sarcoid, TB or other granulomatous disease; infiltration by malignancy
2. Exogenous glucocorticoid therapy	• Suppresses CRF and ACTH secretion

INVESTIGATIONS TO DIFFERENTIATE BETWEEN PRIMARY AND SECONDARY HYPOADRENALISM

These are as follows.

- *Simultaneous measurement of plasma cortisol and ACTH*: ACTH levels are high in Addison's but low or undetectable in secondary adrenal failure. Cortisol levels should also be low.
- *Synacthen test*: In this test, tetracosactrin (Synacthen, which is an ACTH analogue) is given as an intramuscular injection and the adrenal response (that is, plasma cortisol) is measured after a period of time. The short test is used as a screening test and if abnormal it is usual to proceed to the long Synacthen test to confirm the diagnosis and determine whether the adrenal failure is primary or secondary. A normal response to the long test is for the plasma cortisol to peak at 4 h and to show little further increase in the 24 h sample. In secondary adrenal insufficiency the plasma cortisol gradually increases

ENDOCRINOLOGY

throughout the test (owing to gradual recovery of the adrenals from long-term suppression) and the level at 24 h is considerably greater than the level at 4 h. In Addison's disease the plasma cortisol level remains suppressed throughout the test. An alternative method of performing the long Synacthen test is to give Synacthen 1.0 mg daily for three days and to measure the plasma cortisol 6 h after each dose (Table 2.6).

Table 2.6 Synacthen test

	Positive (normal test)
Short Synacthen test: Synacthen 0.25 mg i.m. at time 0. Plasma cortisol measured at 0 and 30 minutes	• Cortisol increase > 200 nmol/L • Peak level > 550 nmol/L
Long Synacthen test: Synacthen 1.0 mg i.m. at time 0. Plasma cortisol measured at 1, 2, 3, 4, 5, 8 and 24 h	• Peak cortisol (> 1000 nmol/L) at 4 h (in 2° adrenal failure level at 24 h is considerably greater than at 4 h and exceeds 690 nmol/L)
or Synacthen 1.0 mg daily for three days. Plasma cortisol measured 6 h after each dose	• Peak cortisol > 1000 nmol/L on day 1. (in 2° adrenal failure there is a gradual increase in cortisol levels and level on day 3 > 690 nmol/L)

Other investigations are to identify the cause and include:

- Anti-adrenal antibodies.
- CT/MRI of pituitary fossa or adrenals (to look for infiltration or calcification). Needle biopsy of the adrenals may also be performed at this time.
- Dynamic pituitary function tests (in secondary adrenal failure) to assess the degree of pituitary reserve.

2.6

a) Secondary adrenal insufficiency.

The response to the ACTH analogue Synacthen progressively improves throughout the long Synacthen test and by the end of the test is near normal. This is characteristic of 2° adrenal insufficiency in which the adrenal glands become unresponsive after prolonged lack of ACTH stimulation.

b) Pituitary insufficiency (lack of ACTH) or abrupt withdrawal of the steroids used to treat the patient's colitis.

c) Plasma ACTH will be low in pituitary failure but high following withdrawal of steroids (continued adrenal suppression means that there is little feedback inhibition of ACTH release).

PITUITARY-THYROID AXIS
2.7

a) Free T3 assay.

b) T3 thyrotoxicosis.

This patient has greatly suppressed TSH production consistent with hyperthyroidism. Her clinical features are also consistent with a diagnosis of hyperthyroidism but the free T4 is normal. However, one must remember that there are two thyroid hormones and it is T3 that is the most metabolically active. In a minority of cases hyperthyroidism is the result of isolated oversecretion of T3.

The causes of hyperthyroidism are shown in Box 2.1. By far the commonest cause is Graves' disease, which is an organ-specific autoimmune disease in which 'thyroid stimulating autoantibodies' bind to the TSH receptor causing thyroid stimulation with consequent diffuse goitre formation and overproducion and oversecretion of thyroid hormones. It is associated with other organ-specific autoimmune diseases such as pernicious anaemia, myasthenia gravis, type 1 diabetes and vitiligo. The thyroid-stimulating antibodies are of the IgG_1 subclass and therefore can cross the placenta producing transient hyperthyroidism in the fetus.

ENDOCRINOLOGY

> **Box 2.1 Causes of hyperthyroidism**
>
> *Most common*
> Graves' disease
> Toxic multinodular goitre
> Solitary toxic nodule (adenoma)
> Thyroiditis
>   Subacute (de Quervain's)
>   Silent (painless)
>   Postpartum
>
> *Other causes*
> TSH-secreting pituitary adenoma
> Inappropriate TSH hypersecretion syndrome
>   (Thyrotrophs of the anterior pituitary are oversensitive to stimulation by TRH)
> Metastatic thyroid carcinoma
> Hydatidiform mole or choriocarcinoma
>   (Excess βHCG secreted by these tumours is able to stimulate the thyroid since βHCG has a degree of TSH-like activity)
> Teratoma containing thyroid tissue (struma ovarii)
> Thyrotoxicosis factitia (covert consumption of thyroid hormones)
> Drugs e.g. amiodarone

INVESTIGATION OF HYPERTHYROIDISM

Investigation is aimed at confirmation of the diagnosis and determining the cause. Confirmation of the diagnosis is by measurement of the individual thyroid hormones (free or total) together with TSH: in thyrotoxicosis levels of the hormones are elevated and TSH is suppressed because of feedback inhibition. Occasionally only T3 is elevated (T3 toxicosis) but TSH will be suppressed. Very rarely both TSH and the thyroid hormones are elevated, in which case the differential diagnosis is between a TSH-secreting pituitary adenoma or inappropriate TSH hypersecretion syndrome (see answer to Q 2.12).

Investigations to determine the cause of hyperthyroidism include:

- *Thyroid ultrasound scan ± fine needle aspiration biopsy*: Ultrasound will demonstrate the presence of a multi-nodular goitre or solitary thyroid nodule. In the case of the latter FNA can be performed to obtain material for cytology.
- *Radioisotope scan of the thyroid*: This will show diffusely increased uptake in Graves' disease; a solitary area of

Table 2.7 Clinical features of hyperthyroidism* and hypothyroidism

Hyperthyroidism	Hypothyroidism
General Heat intolerance, tremor, restlessness, goitre	Lethargy, easy fatiguability, cold intolerance, goitre, pallor, puffy face and hands
Cardiovascular Hypertension, tachycardia, atrial fibrillation, palpitations, heart failure	Bradycardia, heart failure, pericardial/pleural effusions, low voltage ECG complexes
Gastrointestinal Weight loss, ↑ appetite, diarrhoea	Weight gain, loss of appetite, constipation
Genitourinary Oligo/amenorrhoea, loss of libido	Menorrhagia, oligo/amenorrhoea, hyperprolactinaemia (↑TRH stimulates prolactin release)
Ocular Lid lag, lid retraction, ophthalmopathy*	
Dermatological Pretibial myxoedema*, acropachy*, onycholysis, pruritus	Dry skin, dry brittle hair, alopecia
Musculoskeletal Proximal myopathy, fatiguability, hypercalcaemia	Myalgia
Neurological Choreoathetosis	Carpal tunnel syndrome, slow-relaxing reflexes, deafness, cerebellar ataxia, hoarse voice
Haematological Rarely lymphadenopathy or splenomegaly	Anaemia (macrocytic related to thyroid disease or associated pernicious anaemia: microcytic secondary to iron deficiency from menorrhagia)
Psychological Anxiety, irritability, psychosis	Mental slowing, poor concentration, poor memory, depression, pseudodementia, psychosis (myxoedema madness)
Some patients with hyperthyroidism present with lethargy and tiredness (apathetic hyperthyroidism) rather than the classical symptoms. This presentation is more common in elderly patients.	

*These features are only found in Graves' disease

ENDOCRINOLOGY

increased activity (hotspot) with suppression of the surrounding thyroid tissue in the case of a toxic nodule (thyroid carcinoma characteristically, but not always, results in a 'cold spot' surrounded by normal thyroid) and diffusely reduced uptake in the case of subacute or painless thyroiditis (see answer to Q 2.12).
- *Thyroid autoantibodies*: These are not usually necessary in hyperthyroidism but will be present in virtually all cases of Graves' disease and painless thyroiditis. Only the anti-thyroglobulin and anti-microsomal antibodies are routinely measured.
- *TRH stimulation test*: This test is now almost obsolete but you may be asked to interpret the results in an MRCP question. In patients with thyrotoxicosis TSH is suppressed and administration of TRH does not cause elevated TSH levels (flat response). A flat response may also be seen with excess T4 replacement, TSH-secreting pituitary adenomas, and Cushing syndrome (including corticosteroid treatment) but in the latter two conditions the basal TSH should be normal or elevated.

2.8

a) Sick euthyroid syndrome.

b) Repeat the thyroid function tests when the patient is well.

Although the T4 and T3 are low, suggesting hypothyroidism, the TSH is also low. This is inconsistent with primary hypothyroidism. It could be explained by secondary hypothyroidism (caused by inadequate TSH secretion by the anterior pituitary) but this condition is rare. A far more common explanation is the sick euthyroid syndrome.

Severe or chronic illness can affect thyroid function in many ways including reduced concentration of binding proteins; reduced peripheral conversion of T4 to T3 with more rT3 production and reduced TSH production. The sick euthyroid syndrome usually consists of low total and free T4 and T3 together with a normal or low TSH. However, variations on this can occur, for example low T4 but normal T3 (often seen in severe illness such as septicaemia) or low T3 with normal T4 (can be seen in most types of illness, and in 20–30% of geriatric admissions). The common factor is a normal or slightly reduced TSH.

Table 2.8 Causes of hypothyroidism

Primary hypothyroidism
1. Autoimmune (lymphocytic) thyroiditis
   - Female:male = 6:1, peak age 30–50 years
   - Associated with thyroid autoantibodies
   - May be associated with other organ-specific autoimmune diseases

   Two main variants
   Hashimoto's disease
   - Atrophy with regeneration → goitre formation

   Atrophic (idiopathic) thyroiditis
   - No goitre
2. Congenital
   Abnormality/agenesis of thyroid
   Dyshormonogenesis
   - Caused by deficiency of one or more key enzymes for thyroid hormone synthesis
3. Iatrogenic
   Radioiodine
   Thyroidectomy
   Anti-thyroid drugs
   - Post treatment for hyperthyroidism
4. Riedel's thyroiditis
   - Diffuse fibrosis of thyroid and surrounding structures → 'woody' hard goitre. Cause unknown.
5. Endemic goitre
   - Occurs in areas with low environmental iodine levels
   - Most patients just have a goitre with no hypothyroidism
6. Drugs
   Amiodarone
   Lithium
7. Peripheral resistance to thyroid hormone

Secondary hypothyroidism
1. Hypothalamic or pituitary disease
   - For example: pituitary tumours; post pituitary surgery or irradiation; postpartum pituitary haemorrhage (Sheehan syndrome); infiltration by sarcoid, TB or other granulomatous disease; infiltration by malignancy
2. Isolated TSH deficiency

2.9

a) Pregnancy test.

Although the total T4 is high, the TSH is normal indicating that the patient is euthyroid. Fine tremor and tachycardia are non-specific signs and could easily be attributed to anxiety. Vomiting and amenorrhoea are consistent with a diagnosis of pregnancy and pregnancy is associated with an increase in thyroid-binding globulin. The latter causes an increase in total T4 but does not affect the free thyroxine level. Conversely, reduced thyroxine-binding globulin will produce reduced total T4 and T3 levels. Only free thyroxine is biologically active.

Free thyroxine assay would be another acceptable answer but would not be awarded as many marks as the answer above, which will confirm the suspected diagnosis.

Box 2.2 Causes of altered thyroxine-binding globulin (TBG) levels	
↑ TBG	↓ TBG
Familial	Familial
Pregnancy	Androgens
Oestrogen therapy (including oral contraceptive pill)	Cushing
	Thyrotoxicosis
Phenothiazines	Major illness
Hypothyroidism	Malnutrition

2.10

a) Poor compliance.

The patient is only taking her thyroxine for a few days prior to clinic, thus although the free thyroxine level is normal, it has not been normal for long enough to cause suppression of TSH to within the normal range.

2.11

a) Subacute thyroiditis (de Quervain's thyroiditis).

b) Simple analgesia. Systemic steroids can be used if the inflammation is severe.

c) A radioiodine 131 uptake scan will show globally reduced uptake.

In de Quervain's thyroiditis inflammation of the thyroid produces pain and swelling in the neck, and damage to thyroid follicles results in release of preformed thyroid hormones, which may produce transient thyrotoxicosis. This damage also prevents uptake of radioactive iodine during isotope scanning. A high ESR is characteristic. The exact aetiology is unknown, but it is thought to be viral in origin. Recovery is complete and the patient is nearly always left euthyroid, although cases of hypothyroidism following de Quervain's thyroiditis are well documented.

Silent thyroiditis is inflammatory thyroid disorder and can also cause hyperthyroidism with globally reduced uptake on radioactive iodine scanning. However, this condition is autoimmune in origin (associated with thyroid autoantibodies) and is characteristically painless.

2.12

a) TSH-secreting pituitary tumour or inappropriate TSH hypersecretion syndrome.

b) A TRH stimulation test, measurement of TSH glycoprotein α subunit levels or CT/MRI of the pituitary fossa could all be used to determine the correct diagnosis.

This patient has elevated levels of unbound thyroid hormones and biological symptoms that are compatible with a diagnosis of hyperthyroidism. However, one would expect the TSH to be suppressed. Hyperthyroidism may rarely be produced by a TSH-secreting pituitary adenoma or, even more rarely, inappropriate hypersecretion of TSH caused by increased sensitivity of the thyrotroph cells to stimulation by TRH. In the latter syndrome the anterior pituitary remains sensitive to the effects of TRH (which causes further TSH secretion during a TRH test) and bromocriptine (which will suppress TSH secretion). In the case of pituitary adenomas TSH secretion is autonomous and the TSH response to the TRH test is therefore flat.

TSH consists of an α and a β subunit. TSH-secreting pituitary adenomas often secrete excess amounts of α subunits in addition to TSH. This is not the case with inappropriate TSH hypersecretion.

ENDOCRINOLOGY

PITUITARY-GONADAL AXIS

2.13

a) Polycystic ovary syndrome (PCOS).

b) Ovarian ultrasound to demonstrate polycystic ovaries and exclude ovarian carcinoma.

c) Advise her to lose weight if secondary amenorrhoea and hirsutism are the main problems.

This patient presents with secondary amenorrhoea and hirsutism. The causes of these symptoms are shown in Table 2.9 and Box 2.3, respectively. However, the hormonal pattern of elevated LH and testosterone with normal FSH is characteristic of PCOS. Oestrogen levels would be high or normal. Congenital adrenal hyperplasia caused by 21-hydroxylase deficiency is unlikely in the presence of normal 17(OH)-progesterone levels. In the case of virilization as a result of adrenal or ovarian tumours, the testosterone is usually greater than 7 nmol/L (often in the adult male range) and hirsutism develops quickly (over a period of a few months) and is accompanied by other signs of virilization such as deep voice, muscle development and clitoromegaly. The symptoms of PCOS may get worse with obesity and resolve with weight loss.

Box 2.3 Causes of female hirsutism (also acne and male pattern hair loss)
1. Polycystic ovary syndrome (commonest cause)
2. Cushing syndrome
3. 21-hydroxylase deficiency
4. Adrenal tumour
5. Ovarian tumour
6. Idiopathic (5%)

Table 2.9 Causes of primary and secondary amenorrhoea

	Primary amenorrhoea	Secondary amenorrhoea
Always consider		
Pregnancy	+	+
True menopause (if > 40 years)	+	+
Ovarian disease		
Polycystic ovary disease	+	+
Primary ovarian failure	+	+
Resistant ovary syndrome	+	+
Anti-cancer chemotherapy	+	+
Virilizing tumours	+	+
Gonadal dysgenesis (Turner syndrome)	+	+ (if mosaicism present)
Hypothalamic/pituitary disease		
Hypogonadotrophic hypogonadism		
Impaired GnRH secretion	+	+
Impaired LH/FSH secretion	+	+
Kallman syndrome (anosmia and failure to produce GnRH; X-linked)	+	−
Hyperprolactinaemia	+	+
Cushing's disease	+	+
Adrenal disease		
Cushing syndrome	+	+
Virilizing tumours	+	+
21-hydroxylase deficiency	+	+
Thyroid disease		
Hyper- or hypothyroidism	+	+
Other		
Excessive exercise	+	+
Excessive weight loss (e.g. anorexia nervosa)	+	+
Psychological stress	+	+
Congenital abnormalities of genital tract e.g. absent uterus imperforate hymen	+	−
Testicular feminization syndrome (male genotype but female phenotype due to resistance to actions of testosterone)	+	−

2.14

a) Primary ovarian failure (premature menopause = occurrence of menopause before the age of 40).

b) Karyotyping (to exclude Turner syndrome or other abnormalities of sex chromosomes) and laparoscopic ovarian biopsy are indicated.

A normal level of βHCG excludes pregnancy, which should always be considered in someone who has secondary amenorrhoea. In addition, if this woman was pregnant the levels of LH and FSH would be greatly suppressed because of high circulating levels of oestrogens (oestriol mainly) and progesterone from the placenta. The tests show low levels of oestrogen together with greatly elevated gonadotrophins – this is the pattern seen in post-menopausal women. Primary ovarian failure is literally a premature menopause and may be autoimmune in nature since anti-ovarian antibodies are found in about 80% of cases (it is also associated with other organ-specific autoimmune diseases such as Addison's, hypothyroidism and diabetes). Ovarian biopsy would show few or no follicles. There is no curative treatment but affected individuals should be given hormone replacement therapy in view of the risk of osteoporosis caused by oestrogen deficiency.

Another related condition that may come up in the MRCP is 'resistant ovary syndrome'. In this condition there is amenorrhoea and the ovaries appear to be resistant to the effects of gonadotrophins. The biochemical picture is of a normal oestrogen with elevated FSH and LH.

2.15

a) MRI scan of the pituitary fossa, dynamic pituitary function tests and serum prolactin levels are all indicated.

b) Pituitary tumour.

The clear discharge from the nipple is galactorrhoea and is highly suggestive of hyperprolactinaemia. Failure to elevate the gonadotrophins in response to a low serum testosterone level indicates that hypothalamic or pituitary disease is present, which has caused hypogonadotrophic hypogonadism. Thus, either a prolactinoma or a tumour-causing compression of the pituitary stalk (with consequent increased prolactin secretion) are the most likely diagnoses. Despite the normal resting level of TSH it is possible that secretion of other pituitary hormones will also be affected and dynamic pituitary function tests are therefore necessary to assess pituitary reserve.

The causes of hyperprolactinaemia are shown in Box 2.4. Elevated levels of prolactin interfere with the normal pulsatility of GnRH secretion and, to a lesser extent, block the effect of LH on the ovary/testis and can therefore cause hypogonadism even in the absence of pituitary dysfunction.

ENDOCRINOLOGY

Box 2.4 Causes of hyperprolactinaemia

Physiological
1. Pregnancy
2. Suckling (in early stages)
3. Stress
4. Sleep
5. Food (levels rise within 1 h of eating)
6. Nipple stimulation

Drugs
1. Dopamine antagonists
    Phenothiazines
    Butyrophenones
    Thioxanthines
    Metoclopramide
    Sulpiride

2. Dopamine-depleting drugs
    Methyldopa
    Reserpine

3. Hormones
    Oestrogens
    Anti-androgens

4. Opiates
5. Verapamil

Pathological
1. Pituitary prolactinoma
2. Other pituitary tumours secreting prolactin e.g.
    Somatotroph tumours secreting GH and prolactin
    Corticotroph tumours secreting ACTH and prolactin
3. Pituitary tumours causing stalk compression
4. Disease of hypothalamus/pituitary stalk e.g.
    Granulomatous disease e.g. sarcoid
    Craniopharyngioma
    Aneurysm/metastatic cancer causing stalk compression
    Stalk section e.g. following head injury
    Empty sella syndrome
5. Primary hypothyroidism (↑ TRH stimulates prolactin release)
6. Chronic renal failure (caused by both ↑ production and ↓ excretion)
7. Cirrhosis
8. Seizures (prolactin ↑ immediately following seizure and is useful in differentiating true seizures from pseudoseizures)

MINERALOCORTICOID AXIS

2.16

a) Bartter syndrome.

b) Twenty-four hour urine prostaglandin and chloride excretion will be high in Bartter syndrome. Both plasma renin activity and aldosterone levels will also be high in Bartter whereas in primary hyperaldosteronism renin levels will be suppressed by the raised levels of aldosterone. In addition a reduced pressor response to infused angiotensin II (that is, BP will not rise as much as expected) is characteristic of Bartter syndrome.

c) Potassium supplements ± magnesium, potassium-sparing diuretics (amiloride, spironolactone, triamterine) and prostaglandin synthetase inhibitors (typically indomethacin) are all used to treat Bartter syndrome. ACE inhibitors should be avoided since they can precipitate profound hypotension.

Hypokalaemia with urinary potassium wasting is characteristic of excess aldosterone. Normal examination makes most of the causes of secondary hyperaldosteronism unlikely (CCF, cirrhosis, fluid depletion) and normal blood pressure makes primary hyperaldosteronism or renal artery stenosis (another cause of secondary hyperaldosteronism) unlikely. Thus, Bartter syndrome remains as the most likely cause. Hyperglycaemia/diabetes mellitus and hypercalcaemia, which are common causes of polyurea and polydipsia, are excluded by the blood tests.

Bartter syndrome usually presents in childhood with failure to thrive and is characterized by hypokalaemic alkalosis with renal potassium and chloride wasting and normal or low BP (in contrast to primary hyperaldosteronism where the BP is characteristically ↑). Other characteristic features include:

- Hyperplasia of the juxtaglomerular apparatus
- Hypersecretion of prostaglandins → ↑ urinary prostaglandin excretion (may also → inhibition of platelet function)
- High plasma renin activity → hyperaldosteronism.

Bartter syndrome is thought to be caused by abnormal chloride transport in the thick ascending limb of the loop of Henle.

ENDOCRINOLOGY

> **Box 2.5 Causes of hypokalaemia**
>
> **↑ K⁺ loss**
> *Renal*
> 1°/2°/3° hyperaldosteronism
> Cushing syndrome
> Bartter syndrome
> Congenital adrenal hyperplasia
> Renin-secreting tumour (→ ↑ aldosterone)
> Renal tubular acidosis
> Drugs
>   Diuretic abuse
>   Carbonic anhydrase inhibitors (→ renal tubular acidosis)
>   Liquorice/carbenoxolone (inhibit 11β hydroxysteroid dehydrogenase
>   Amphotericin B, gentamicin, amikacin
> Diuretic phase of acute tubular necrosis
> Acute leukaemias
> Alkalosis
>
> *Gastrointestinal tract*
> Diarrhoea/purgative abuse
> Vomiting (particularly with pyloric stenosis)
> Enteric fistula
> Rectal villous adenoma
> Ileostomy
> Ureterosigmoidostomy (→ renal tubular acidosis)
>
> **ECF to ICF shift**
> Alkalosis
> ↑ Catecholamines (e.g. post MI)
> Insulin
> Familial hypokalaemic periodic paralysis

2.17

a) Primary hyperaldosteronism.

The clinical picture of hypertension with hypokalaemic alkalosis is highly suggestive of mineralocorticoid excess. Cushing syndrome can produce a similar picture, especially when caused by ectopic ACTH, but this is unlikely in the presence of a normal glucose tolerance test (for interpretation of the GTT see answer to Q 2.24). One would not expect the patient to be hypernatraemic in the presence of secondary hyperaldosteronism unless he were volume depleted (for example by congestive cardiac failure or cirrhosis). Thus, primary hyperaldosteronism remains as the most likely cause.

b) Measure paired plasma renin and aldosterone levels under conditions of salt loading or following plasma expansion with a normal saline infusion (1.25 litres over 2 h or 2 litres over 4 h; done between 8 a.m. and noon).

c) Aldosterone-secreting adrenal adenoma (Conn syndrome) or bilateral adrenal hyperplasia.

d) Any of the following tests can be used. However, imaging is not usually performed until a biochemical diagnosis has been made because a large number of non-functioning adenomas are found incidentally when the adrenals are imaged. Adrenal vein catheterization is the most sensitive test but is not without risk and is therefore usually reserved for cases where results of the other tests have been inconclusive.

- Measure aldosterone levels supine and then after standing for 4 h – in Conn syndrome the aldosterone levels remain unchanged or, paradoxically, fall. In adrenal hyperplasia they rise on standing as is the case in normal individuals.
- Measure the aldosterone response to an angiotensin II infusion – flat response (i.e. no increase) in Conn but aldosterone levels increase in response to angiotensin II in adrenal hyperplasia.
- Measure plasma or 24 h urinary 18-oxocortisone or 18-hydroxycortisone. This is raised in adrenal adenoma; normal or less raised in idiopathic adrenal hyperplasia.
- CT or MRI scan of adrenals may show adenoma or bilateral enlargement (in hyperplasia).
- Radiolabelled iodocholesterol or radiolabelled 6β[^{131}I]-iodomethyl-19-norcholesterol scan after treatment with dexamethasone for six weeks shows unilateral uptake in Conn's adenoma but bilateral uptake in hyperplasia.
- Selective blood sampling from adrenal veins; increased aldosterone levels are found on the side of an adenoma with reduced or supressed levels on the other side (diagnosis of adrenal adenoma requires aldosterone levels on one side to be ten times that on the other side). Aldosterone levels are elevated in blood samples from both sides in adrenal hyperplasia. Blood is usually also sampled from the IVC as a reference.

ENDOCRINOLOGY

Table 2.10 Causes of primary hyperaldosteronism

	Response of aldosterone to various stimuli				Other features
	Upright posture	Ag II infusion	ACE inhibitor	Dex. suppression	

1. Adrenal adenoma (70%)
  Conn's adenoma
  Angiotensin II
  responsive adenoma
	→/↓
	
	↑
		→/↓
		
		↑
			→
			
			↓
				→
				
				→
					18-oxocortisol and 18-hydroxycortisol also produced in excess

2. Idiopathic adrenal hyperplasia (rarely unilateral) (30%)	↑	↑	↓	→	
3. Primary adrenal hyperplasia	→/↓	→/↓	→	→	
4. Glucocorticoid-suppressible hyperaldosteronism	→/↓	→/↓	→	↓	18-oxocortisol and 18-hydroxycortisol also produced in excess
5. Aldosterone-producing adrenal carcinoma (rare)	→	→	→	→	Other steroids (androgens, oestrogens, cortisol) often produced in excess as well

2.18

a) Congenital adrenal hyperplasia (CAH) caused by 21-hydroxylase deficiency.

b) Androgen-secreting adrenal carcinoma or testicular carcinoma secreting testosterone (Leydig cell tumour) or βHCG.

c) Elevated plasma 17-hydroxyprogesterone or urinary pregnanetrione are highly suggestive of congenital adrenal hyperplasia. Ultrasound or CT of adrenals and ultrasound of the testes to exclude a tumour are also indicated.

The causes of precocious puberty are shown in Table 2.11. This child's premature virilization is being caused by elevated levels of serum testosterone, but the pre-pubertal testicular size makes premature activation of the hypothalamic-pituitary system unlikely. Normal testicular examination, although not excluding testicular carcinoma, makes it less likely. Adrenal

Table 2.11 Causes of precocious puberty and female virilization

	Boys	Girls	
	Precocious puberty	Precocious puberty	Virilization
Congenital adrenal hyperplasia			
21-hydroxylase deficiency	+	−	+
11β-hydroxylase deficiency	+	−	+
3β-hydroxysteroid dehydrogenase deficiency	−	−	+
Testicular tumours			
Leydig cell (secretes testosterone)	+	−	−
βHCG secreting	+	−	−
Ovarian tumours			
Usually caused by Sertoli-theca cell tumours (secrete oestrogen), but other tumours that secrete oestrogens (or androgens that can be converted to oestrogens by peripheral tissues) may be the cause	−	+	+
Adrenal tumours			
Generally androgen-secreting tumours cause precocious puberty in males and virilization in females whilst oestrogen-secreting tumours cause precocious puberty in females. However some adrenal tumours secreting weak androgens can cause precocious puberty in females by peripheral conversion to oestrogens	+	+	+
Premature activation of the hypothalamic-pituitary axis			
Idiopathic	+	+	−
Due to underlying CNS abnormality e.g. tumour	+	+	−
Other causes			
Primary hypothyroidism (↑TRH stimulates FSH secretion causing ovarian oestrogen production)	−	+	−
McCune–Albright syndrome	−	+	−
Russell–Silver syndrome	−	+	−
Oestrogen-containing creams and medications	−	+	−

tumours tend to secrete mineralocorticoids and glucocorticoids in addition to androgens. If this were the case one would expect this child to show biochemical signs of mineralocorticoid excess, that is, hypokalaemia and hypernatraemia (or borderline-high sodium). In fact there is evidence of mineralocorticoid deficiency (hyponatraemia and slightly high potassium), which is further evidence of 21-hydroxylase deficiency.

CALCIUM METABOLISM

Approximately 50% of serum calcium is bound to albumin, the remainder being free-ionized calcium. Since it is only the free calcium that is 'active' assays of total calcium have to be interpreted together with the serum albumin concentration. A useful formula to correct the total calcium for the albumin concentration is as follows:

$$[Ca]_{corrected} = [Ca]_{measured} + 0.02 (40 - [Alb]_{measured})$$

where $[Ca]_{measured}$ = the measured serum calcium concentration and $[Alb]_{measured}$ = the measured serum albumin concentration.

A useful rule of thumb is that calcium and phosphate concentrations always change in opposite directions unless renal failure or vitamin D deficiency is present. This is illustrated by Table 2.12.

Table 2.12 Biochemical abnormalities seen in various disorders of bone/calcium metabolism

	Calcium	Phosphate	ALP
1°/3° hyperparathyroidism	↑	↓	↑/→
2° hyperparathyroidism	↓/→	↓	↑/→
Hypo/pseudohypoparathyroisism	↓	↑	→
Osteomalacia	↓	↓	↑
Osteoporosis	→	→	→
Multiple myeloma	↑	↑/→	→
Paget's disease[†]	→	→	↑↑
Multiple bony metastases	↑	↑/→	↑
Chronic renal failure	↓	↑	↑/→

[†] Hypercalcaemia may occur in Paget's patients that are immobile

2.19

See also questions 2.24, 2.25, 8.1 and 8.4

a) A blood glucose level should always be measured following a seizure.

b) Hypoparathyroidism, pseudohypoparathyroidism and severe magnesium deficiency.

Chronic renal failure, hypoparathyroidism and pseudohypoparathyroidism are the conditions that produce this biochemical picture. However, in this case the renal function is normal. Severe magnesium deficiency impairs parathyroid hormone release and therefore also needs to be excluded. In pseudohypoparathyroidism the cells are resistant to the effects of PTH resulting in the same biochemical abnormalities as hypoparathyroidism but with a high PTH (since low calcium stimulates PTH secretion). Pseudohypoparathyroidism is a familial condition, which is inherited in an X-linked dominant fashion. It is also associated with a number of physical characteristics including a round face and short metatarsal and metacarpal bones.

In this case the seizure was probably caused by hypocalcaemia.

c) Measure (i) serum parathyroid hormone level (since this will be low in hypoparathyroidism and normal or high in pseudohypoparathyroidism); (ii) serum magnesium level; and (iii) urinary phosphate and cyclic AMP following a parathyroid hormone infusion. The latter test will show a normal response (increased urinary phosphate and cAMP) in hypoparathyroidism but an abnormal response in pseudohypoparathyroidism. The type of abnormality seen can be used to characterize the form of pseudohypoparathyroidism that is present: patients in which neither urinary phosphate nor cAMP is increased are classified as type I pseudohypoparathyroidism and those in which urinary cAMP only rises are classed as type II.

d) Hypocalcaemia produces a prolonged QT interval.

ENDOCRINOLOGY

> **Box 2.6 Causes of hypocalcaemia**
>
> 1. Chronic renal failure
>   Caused by a combination of reduced $1,25(OH)_2VitD_3$ synthesis and increased serum phosphate (exceeds solubility product for calcium phosphate → reduced ionized calcium)
> 2. Hypoparathyroidism
>   Post-thyroid surgery
>   Idiopathic (autoimmune)
>   Severe hypomagnesaemia
>   Congenital e.g. DiGeorge syndrome
> 3. Pseudohypoparathyroidism
> 4. Vitamin D deficiency
>   Dietary
>   Vitamin D-dependent rickets type I
> 5. Vitamin D resistance (vitamin D-dependent rickets type II)
> 6. Malabsorption
> 7. Drugs
>   Prolonged use of anti-convulsants (especially phenytoin and phenobarbitone)
>   Phosphate therapy
>   Calcitonin
>   Diphosphonates
> 8. Artefact e.g. low serum albumin concentration
> 9. Miscellaneous
>   Acute pancreatitis
>   Prostate cancer

2.20

a) Serum amylase. A level > 1000 U/ml is highly suggestive, if not diagnostic, of acute pancreatitis.

b) Acute pancreatitis secondary to hypercalcaemia.

c) Primary hyperparathyroidism or bony metastases (Box 2.7) are the commonest causes of hypercalcaemia, but the presence of a low serum phosphate and low bicarbonate (acidosis) make primary hyperparathyroidism most likely. Other causes of hypercalcaemia are shown in Box 2.8.

d) Assay for parathyroid hormone and a bone scan are indicated. The patient should also be screened for multiple myeloma (ESR, serum immunoglobulins, paraproteins and urinary Bence-Jones protein) since this would be the next most common cause of hypercalcaemia of this magnitude. A hydrocortisone suppression test could also be performed (10 days hydrocortisone 40 mg t.d.s. → serum calcium levels classically do not suppress in primary hyperparathyroidism whereas they do in other causes of hypercalcaemia). However, many would regard this test as obsolete now that sensitive assays for PTH are available. It may still come up as a data interpretation question though.

The patient's symptoms are strongly suggestive of pancreatitis and the bruising around the umbilicus is Cullen's sign, which classically occurs in this condition. Bruising of the flanks (Turner's sign) may also be seen. Hypercalcaemia is a well recognized precipitant of pancreatitis and the low serum phosphate together with metabolic acidosis indicate that excess PTH is the likely cause. Hyperchloraemic metabolic acidosis is characteristic of primary hyperparathyroidism whereas hypochloraemic metabolic alkalosis is more characteristic of bony metastases.

Box 2.7 Tumours that metastasize to bone

1. Bronchus
2. Breast
3. Thyroid
4. Renal
5. Prostate (most prostate bony mets do not cause hypercalcaemia since they are osteosclerotic rather than osteolytic)
6. Ovary
7. Bowel (rarely)

Some tumours are capable of secreting a PTH-related peptide (PTHrP), which causes the same biochemical picture as primary hyperparathyroidism but these are rare and modern immunoassays for PTH should be able to discriminate between PTH and PTHrP. Squamous cell carcinoma of the bronchus is the commonest source of ectopic PTHrP (other tumours include renal, bladder, breast, ovary, pancreas and lymphoma).

ENDOCRINOLOGY

Box 2.8 Causes of hypercalcaemia

1. Primary*/tertiary hyperparathyroidism
2. Malignancy*
    Bony metastases
    Myeloma
    PTHrP-secreting tumour
3. Familial hypocalcuric hypercalcaemia
4. Sarcoidosis (and other granulomatous disease)
    (1α-hydroxylation of 25(OH)VitD$_3$ to 1,25(OH)$_2$VitD$_3$ by granuloma macrophages)
5. Vitamin D intoxication*
6. Hyperthyroidism
7. Phaeochromocytoma
8. Addison's disease
9. Acute renal failure
10. Thiazide diuretics
11. Milk-alkali syndrome
12. Artefact e.g. high serum albumin concentration

*Main causes of severe hypercalcaemia

2.21

a) Vitamin D-resistant rickets (hypophosphataemic rickets).

b) Measure 24 h urinary phosphate excretion, which will be high in this condition (not specific though). Vitamin D and PTH levels will be normal.

c) Phosphate supplementation is most important, together with calcitriol.

The X-ray changes are characteristic of rickets and the elevated ALP and skeletal deformity are compatible with this diagnosis, but the serum calcium is normal. The clue to the correct diagnosis lies in the serum phosphate level, which is low, indicating that vitamin D-resistant rickets is the probable diagnosis. This condition is inherited in an X-linked dominant fashion and usually presents in infancy or childhood with failure to thrive. It is caused by impaired renal-tubular reabsorption of phosphate, which results in marked hypophosphataemia. The changes of rickets (or osteomalacia in adults) are caused by the hypophosphataemia rather than vitamin D deficiency and the serum calcium, PTH and vitamin D levels are therefore usually normal. ALP is elevated.

Treatment with vitamin D alone has very little effect but the addition of phosphate supplementation reverses the skeletal abnormalities if given early enough.

Vitamin D-dependent rickets is another familial disorder of vitamin D metabolism. There are two types: type I is inherited in an autosomal recessive fashion and is caused by impaired renal 1α-hydroxylation of 25(OH)-cholecalciferol. Tissue responsiveness to calcitriol (1,25(OH)$_2$VitD) is normal and this condition therefore responds well to calcitriol replacement therapy. Type II is inherited in an autosomal dominant fashion and is caused by a defect in the vitamin D receptor, which makes the tissues resistant to calcitriol. Calcitriol levels are usually normal.

GUT HORMONES

2.22

a) Self-administration of insulin/sulphonylureas and insulinoma are the most likely differential diagnoses.

b) Measurement of paired insulin, C-peptide and glucose levels during a period of fasting.

The causes of fasting hypoglycaemia are shown in Table 2.13. By far the most likely diagnoses are insulinoma or self-administration of insulin/sulphonylurea drugs – the latter diagnosis should always be suspected in health-care workers who present with fasting hypoglycaemia.

During insulin release proinsulin is cleaved to form insulin and C-peptide, both of which are released into the circulation in equimolar proportions. Insulin secretion by insulinomas is autonomous and diagnosis of an insulinoma relies upon demonstrating high levels of insulin and C-peptide in the presence of a low blood glucose, for example during a period of fasting. In contrast, hypoglycaemia associated with self-administration of insulin will be accompanied by high insulin levels but low C-peptide (caused by suppression of endogenous insulin secretion). Sulphonylurea drugs (which stimulate insulin secretion by the pancreas) produce the same pattern of insulin and C-peptide levels as an insulinoma but can be differentiated by measurement of plasma or urinary sulphonylurea levels.

ENDOCRINOLOGY

Table 2.13 Causes of fasting hypoglycaemia

	Comment
1. Insulinoma	
2. Self-administration of insulin/sulphonylureas	
3. Alcohol	Alcohol metabolism is at the expense of hepatic gluconeogenesis and in alcoholics hypoglycaemia can therefore develop during prolonged fasting, when glycogen stores are exhausted. Children are particularly susceptible because of faster glucose turnover.
4. Addison's disease	
5. Pituitary insufficiency	Impaired secretion of both growth hormone and ACTH required for hypoglycaemia in adults. Impaired secretion of either hormone is sufficient to produce hypoglycaemia in children.
6. Liver failure	Impaired gluconeogenesis and glycolysis.
7. Non-pancreatic tumours	Most commonly retroperitoneal sarcomas. These secrete insulin-like growth factor 2, which activates the insulin receptor.
8. Autoimmune hypoglycaemia (e.g. in Hodgkin's)	
Insulin receptor antibodies	These normally cause insulin-resistant diabetes by blocking the insulin receptor. Rarely they cause receptor activation with fasting hypoglycaemia.
Anti-insulin antibodies	These may cause accumulation of antibody-bound insulin, which then dissociates resulting in high insulin levels.

Additional causes to consider in infants/children

1. Nesidioblastosis	Congenital abnormality with overgrowth of pancreatic β-islet cells. Produces persistent hypoglycaemia from birth.
2. von Gierke's disease	Glycogen storage disease caused by glucose-6-phosphatase deficiency.
3. Galactosaemia	Caused by galactose-1-phosphate uridyl transferase deficiency.
4. Fructose intolerance	Caused by fructose-6-phosphate aldolase deficiency. Hypoglycaemia occurs when fructose introduced into the diet (~ 6 months).

2.23

a) 24 h urinary 5-hydroxyindole acetic acid (5HIAA).

b) Carcinoid syndrome (carcinoid tumour).

This patient has developed right-heart failure on a backgound of chronic diarrhoea and episodes of wheezing. The presence of CV waves on clinical examination is indicative of tricuspid regurgitation. The cardiac catheter data are normal apart from a mildly elevated right atrial pressure, which is due to tricuspid regurgitation. This excludes pulmonary hypertension, pulmonary stenosis, mitral stenosis and left-to-right shunting of blood (in other words, all the usual causes) as causes of the right-sided heart failure. Normal bronchoscopy and normal lung function tests make primary lung disease an unlikely cause for the attacks of wheezing. Carcinoid syndrome classically presents with episodes of flushing and wheeze and is associated with diarrhoea and endocardial fibrosis of the right side of the heart, which typically produces tricuspid regurgitation and may result in right-heart failure.

MULTIPLE ENDOCRINE ABNORMALITIES

2.24

a) Impaired glucose tolerance, acromegaly and hyperparathyroidism.

b) The pancreas.

c) Multiple endocrine neoplasia type 1 (MEN-1).

The glucose tolerance test should be interpreted as shown in Table 2.14. Based on these criteria the patient has impaired glucose tolerance. Growth hormone (GH) is normally suppressed by rising glucose levels and one would therefore expect the GH level to fall during the course of a glucose tolerance test. In this case the growth hormone paradoxically rises. This GH response is characteristically seen in acromegaly (although failure of the GH to suppress would also be suggestive of acromegaly) but it may also be seen in other conditions, including Wilson's disease, heroin addiction and renal failure. In addition the calcium is elevated and the serum phosphate is low, a pattern suggestive of hyperparathyroidism: parathyroid hormone causes reabsorption of calcium from bones (producing hypercalcaemia) and increased renal tubular secretion of phosphate (producing a low or borderline low serum phosphate level).

Table 2.14 Interpretation of glucose tolerance test (75 g oral glucose load)

Glucose measurement (mmol/L)	Normal	Impaired glucose tolerance	Diabetes mellitus
Baseline fasting plasma (blood) glucose	< 7.8* (< 6.7) and	< 7.8† (< 6.7) and	> 7.8† (> 6.7) and/or
2 h plasma (blood) glucose	< 7.8 (< 6.7)	7.8 < glucose < 11.1 (6.7 < glucose < 10.0)	> 11.1 (> 10.0)

*This value is likely to change to 6.0 mmol/L in line with American Diabetic Association criteria
†This value is likely to change to 7.0 mmol/L in line with American Diabetic Association criteria

Hypersecretion of more than one hormone should always raise suspicion of one of the multiple endocrine neoplasia syndromes. In this case the pattern of endocrine abnormality suggests MEN-1, which characteristically involves the pituitary and parathyroid glands and pancreas. Pituitary and parathyroid involvement have already been established so it only remains to demonstrate involvement of the pancreas. The presence of a past history of recurrent duodenal ulcers may be indicative of the presence of a gastrin-secreting tumour (Zollinger–Ellison syndrome). These normally arise in the pancreas and would therefore be consistent with the diagnosis of MEN-1. Measurement of serum gastrin (high) and CT scan of the pancreas should be performed.

Table 2.15 Typical endocrine involvement in multiple endocrine neoplasia

	MEN-1	MEN-2
Parathyroid	Involved in 95% of cases Hyperplastic glands	Involved in 60% of cases Hyperplastic glands (hypercalcaemia only ocurs in ~ 20%)
Pancreas	Involved in 70% of cases Gastrinoma (60%) Insulinoma (30%) VIP, glucagon, somatastatin-secreting or carcinoid tumours rare	
Pituitary	Involved in 50% of cases Prolactinoma (65%) Acromegaly (30%) ACTH	
Thyroid		Involved in ~ 100% of cases Medullary cell carcinoma
Adrenal		Phaeochromocytoma in 50% (70% bilateral) Cushing syndrome *Additional features found in MEN-2B* Marfanoid habitus and mucosal neuromata (especially eyelids, lips and tongue)

2.25

a) Excess parathyroid hormone as a result of parathyroid hyperplasia.

b) Multiple endocrine neoplasia type 2a.

c) Measure urinary vanillylmandelic acid (VMA) and metanephrines or plasma catecholamine levels to screen for phaeochromocytoma and measure plasma calcitonin levels following stimulation with pentagastrin to screen for medullary cell carcinoma of the thyroid. This patient should also have a thyroid ultrasound.

d) Intravenous phentolamine (an α-blocker) or labetalol (a combined α- and β-blocker) to control the blood pressure since this patient may be having a hypertensive crisis.

ENDOCRINOLOGY

The commonest presenting features of a phaeochromocytoma are hypertension, headache and sweating and the latter symptoms often occur in episodes that correspond to periodic surges of catecholamine release (this patient has had two previous episodes). Other evidence that this patient has excess catecholamine production are tachycardia, hyperglycaemia and hypokalaemia (catecholamines promote potassium uptake by cells). This patient also has a mass palpable in the thyroid and although thyrotoxicosis secondary to an overactive nodule could cause tachycardia, hypertension and hypercalcaemia it would not account for the hyperglycaemia or for the patient's strong family history of thyroidectomy. The latter feature is strongly suggestive of a familial syndrome and medullary cell carcinoma of the thyroid is familial (autosomal dominant) in 20% of cases. The combination of phaeochromocytoma and medullary cell carcinoma of the thyroid is known as multiple endocrine neoplasia type 2 (see answer to Q 2.24). Parathyroid hyperplasia is also found in 60% of cases but is not necessary for the diagnosis.

2.26

a) ECG, CK-MB isoenzyme, free thyroxine and TSH, plasma cortisol and blood gases (to exclude diabetic ketoacidosis). CT pituitary fossa, dexamethasone suppression test and thyroid autoantibodies would probably not be done as emergency investigations.

b) Panhypopituitarism with adrenal and/or hypothyroid crisis.

c) The following measures are necessary:

- Intravenous colloid to raise blood pressure.
- Intravenous hydrocortisone followed by cautious administration of intravenous tri-iodothyronine. (Giving tri-iodothyronine without hydrocortisone may precipitate/worsen adrenal crisis in a combined deficiency.)
- Intravenous dextrose.
- Broad-spectrum antibiotics.
- Gradual rewarming.
- Exclude myocardial infarction (as AST is elevated).

The information given suggests that more than one endocrine deficiency is present:

- Slow relaxing reflexes imply hypothyroidism. This diagnosis is supported by the presence of a mild macrocytic anaemia together with raised AST and LDH (AST, LDH and CK may all be elevated in hypothyroidism). The presence of normal albumin and bilirubin means that liver disease is unlikely to be the cause of the elevated enzyme levels. Hypothyroidism can also cause hyponatraemia as a result of the syndrome of inappropriate ADH secretion.
- Loss of libido suggests failure of gonadotrophin secretion.
- Low sodium, anaemia, raised urea, hypotension and hypoglycaemia suggest failure of glucocorticoid production (hypoglycaemia requires that both growth hormone and ACTH secretion are affected).

All of these endocrine failures can be explained by panhypopituitarism with loss of TSH, GnRH and ACTH. Pallor is said to be characteristic of panhypopituitarism.

An alternative diagnosis would be polyglandular deficiency type II (Schmidt syndrome) but this condition is rare. Polyglandular deficiency syndrome is said to have occurred when several organ specific autoimmune endocrine failures occur simultaneously. There are two main types:

- Polyglandular deficiency type I is the combination of Addison's disease, hypoparathyroidism, primary gonadal failure and chronic mucocutaneous candidiasis.
- Polyglandular deficiency type II is the combination of Addison's disease, primary hypothyroidism, primary hypogonadism, insulin-dependent diabetes mellitus, pernicious anaemia and vitiligo.

3 HAEMATOLOGY

3.1

See also questions 5.2, 7.3, and 8.3–8.5

a) Cold agglutinin mediated autoimmune haemolytic anaemia following a viral infection (most commonly EBV or CMV).
b) Haemoglobinuria caused by intravascular haemolysis.

Anaemia with a raised reticulocyte count implies haemolysis. The presence of normal liver enzyme levels means that hepatic dysfunction is unlikely to be the cause of the elevated bilirubin and absence of bilirubin in the urine indicates that the hyperbilirubinaemia is unconjugated (excess bilirubin produced by haemolysis overloads hepatic conjugating capacity resulting in elevated plasma unconjugated bilirubin). Raised urinary urobilinogen is the result of absorption of excess bilinogens (produced by the action of gastrointestinal bacteria on bilirubin) from the gut and subsequent excretion in the urine.

Box 3.1 Causes of cold agglutinins

Primary

1. Chronic cold agglutinin disease
2. Chronic idiopathic paroxysmal nocturnal haemoglobinuria

Secondary

1. Infections
    Mycoplasma pneumoniae
    Syphilis (including congenital) associated with paroxysmal nocturnal haemoglobinuria
    Infective endocarditis
    Legionnaire's disease
    Viruses e.g. EBV, CMV, HIV, influenza, VZV, rubella, mumps
2. Neoplasms
    Waldenström's macroglobulinaemia
    Lymphoma
    Myeloma
    CLL
    Kaposi's sarcoma
3. Autoimmune diseases

3.2

a) Polycythaemia and microcytic anaemia.

b) Polycythaemia rubra vera (now called primary proliferative polycythaemia) with chronic gastrointestinal blood loss resulting in iron deficiency anaemia.

c) Pulmonary embolus (PE) caused by prothrombotic tendency.

d) Appropriate investigations include red cell mass and plasma volume (to confirm true polycythaemia); serum ferritin (a measure of iron stores; serum iron and/or TIBC could also be measured but are not as good); upper GI endoscopy (to look for site of blood loss); and arterial blood gases (to exclude hypoxia as a cause for the polycythaemia). Additional investigations might include neutrophil alkaline phosphatase (raised in PCRV but normal in CGL); renal ultrasound/IVU (to exclude a renal cause for the polycythaemia); and liver ultrasound (to exclude hepatocellular carcinoma). Bone marrow examination is not usually required to diagnose PCRV.

e) Hyperviscosity syndrome or TIAs (polycythaemia is a hypercoagulable state). Other causes of hyperviscosity syndrome include CGL and paraproteinaemias such as Waldenström's macroglobulinaemia and multiple myeloma (especially IgG myeloma).

The MCH and MCHC are low indicating that the patient is actually anaemic despite the normal Hb. A normal Hb in the presence of anaemia should always raise the suspicion of myeloproliferative disorder. In this patient the elevated haematocrit and relatively elevated RCC suggest PCRV (although the RCC is normal, it is actually elevated relative to the degree of anaemia and microcytosis). The WCC (caused by neutrophilia) and platelet count are also usually raised in PCRV, and the Vitamin B_{12} binding proteins may also be high. In addition the basophil count is also often elevated in myeloproliferative disorders. Chronic gastrointestinal blood loss is common in myeloproliferative disorders because of abnormal platelet function causing impaired haemostasis. Paradoxically such patients may also be prothrombotic and can therefore present with both haemorrhagic and thromboembolic events. In this man the latter has resulted in a PE. Thromboses in the microcirculation of the gut may result in frank gastric or duodenal ulceration, which can cause further GI blood loss.

Box 3.2 Causes of polycythaemia

Primary
1. Primary proliferative polycythaemia (polycythaemia rubra vera)
2. Familial erythrocytosis

Secondary
1. Compensatory ↑ in erythropoietin
    Lung disease (hypoxia)
    Heavy smoking
    Haemoglobinopathy with increased affinity haemoglobin
    Cyanotic congenital heart disease
    High altitude living
2. Inappropriate ↑ in erythropoietin
    Renal disease: for example renal cell carcinoma, renal adenoma, renal cysts (solitary or polycystic), Wilms' tumour, hydronephrosis, renal transplant, Bartter syndrome
    Hepatocellular carcinoma, hepatic metastases
    Adrenal tumours: Cushing syndrome, phaeochromocytoma, Conn syndrome
    Massive uterine fibroids/uterine leiomyoma
    Cerebellar haemangioblastoma
3. Relative polycythaemia
    Dehydration: from persistent vomiting, severe diarrhoea, post operatively
    Plasma loss e.g. burns
    Stress polycythaemia (Gaisböck syndrome: found particularly in obese middle-aged men who are hypertensive and smoke)

3.3

a) β thalassaemia trait (carrier state).

b) $\alpha:\beta$ chain synthesis ratio studies (normally 1:1) and serum ferritin.

c) The partner should be screened for thalassaemia trait (and other haemoglobinopathies) so that appropriate genetic counselling can be given.

The thalassaemias are characterized by reduced synthesis of normal globin chains and are mainly divided into α and β types dependent upon the globin chain whose synthesis is affected. Reduced production of one of the globin chains results in reduced synthesis of normal adult haemoglobin ($\alpha_2\beta_2$) and, consequently, anaemia develops. In α thalassaemia the anaemia is present both in utero and after birth as a result of reduced ability to synthesize both fetal haemoglobin ($\alpha_2\delta_2$) and adult haemoglobin, whereas in β thalassaemia anaemia develops at about six months when fetal haemoglobin production is 'switched off'. The severity of the anaemia varies with the degree of reduction of haemoglobin chain synthesis.

In thalassaemia trait (the carrier state) the red blood cells are often microcytic and hypochromic with reduced MCH, mimicking iron deficiency. There is also frequently a mild degree of anaemia, which further confuses the picture. Serum iron, serum ferritin and bone marrow iron stores are however normal. In addition, HbA$_2$ is characteristically raised in β thalassaemia trait. The iron status should be checked and corrected before measuring HbA$_2$ since iron deficiency may result in a falsely low (that is, normal) HbA$_2$.

3.4

a) Red cell folate, serum B$_{12}$ and blood film with staining for reticulocytes are all indicated. On the blood film, hypersegmented neutrophils would be characteristic of megaloblastic anaemia while reticulocytosis would be characteristic of haemolytic anaemia (haemolytic anaemia can produce an apparent macrocytosis owing to the fact that immature red cells released into the circulation are larger than their mature counterparts). Bone marrow aspirate and trephine biopsy is usually unnecessary for the diagnosis of megaloblastic anaemia, but would show megaloblastic erythroblasts (delayed condensation of nuclear chromatin) and giant metamyelocytes.

b) Folate deficiency with megaloblastic anaemia as a result of treatment with phenytoin.

c) Osteomalacia may also occur with phenytoin treatment so this patient may have an associated proximal myopathy.

Folate and/or vitamin D deficiency may occur in patients who are on anti-convulsant medication. The exact mechanism is unknown but it may be because of increased metabolism of the vitamins as a result of induction of cytochrome p450 enzymes by the drug. In this case the serum transaminases are elevated owing to induction.

3.5

a) Chronic lymphocytic leukaemia.

b) Warm antibody autoimmune haemolytic anaemia and hypogammaglobulinaemia.

c) The following investigations are all appropriate:
- Bone marrow aspirate and trephine biopsy with immunophenotyping of infiltrating lymphocytes.
- Direct Coombs' anti-globin test to demonstrate autoimmune haemolytic anaemia.
- Reticulocyte count.
- Serum immunoglobulins.

d) Smear cells are characteristic of CLL.

Polychromasia on the blood film is caused by the presence of increased reticulocytes and, in the presence of anaemia, this strongly suggests haemolysis. Lymphocytosis with autoimmune haemolysis could of course be a result of viral infection such as EBV/CMV, but recurrent chest infection implies immune-paresis and, in a person of this age, CLL is the most likely diagnosis. This can be confirmed by the presence of at least 40% infiltration of the bone marrow by mature lymphocytes, and immunophenotyping can be used to demonstrate monoclonality. Warm antibody AIHA may occur in 15% and anti-platelet antibodies resulting in thrombocytopenia in 5%. Both hypogammaglobulinaemia and myelosuppression from bone marrow infiltration may result in recurrent infection.

3.6

a) The presence of a lupus anti-coagulant.

Failure of the clotting abnormality to correct following addition of normal plasma indicates the presence of an inhibitor of coagulation rather than a clotting factor deficiency. Co-existent deep venous thrombosis (the cause of this patient's swollen calf) makes lupus anti-coagulant likely.

Anti-phospholipid antibodies can be broadly divided into lupus anti-coagulants and anti-cardiolipin antibodies and a number of different anti-phospholipid antibodies of both IgG and IgM subclasses have been described. The lupus anti-coagulant gives rise to a hypercoagulable state (by inhibiting factor X activation) whilst paradoxically prolonging the KPTT (being an anti-phospholipid antibody it effects those tests of coagulation which are dependent on phospholipid such as the KPTT). It was first described in association with systemic lupus erythematosus but it can occur in a wide variety of autoimmune conditions or de novo. Anti-cardiolipin antibodies also predispose to thrombosis but they do not prolong the clotting time. The anti-phospholipid antibody (Hughes) syndrome comprises recurrent miscarriages, and arterial or venous thromboses together with laboratory evidence of a persistent anti-phospholipid antibody (either lupus anti-coagulant or anti-cardiolipin). Mild thrombocytopenia, heart valve disease, livido reticularis, chorea and transient ischaemic attacks may also occur.

Anti-phospholipid antibodies may also cause a false positive VDRL.

3.7

a) Von Willebrand's disease.

b) The main investigations used to diagnose VWD are:
- Ristocetin-induced platelet aggregation.
- Assay for von Willebrand factor (old nomenclature: factor VIII related antigen [VIIIR:Ag]).
- Assay for factor VIII clotting activity (VIIIc).

Von Willebrand's disease (VWD) is an autosomal dominant condition in which there is reduced synthesis of von Willebrand factor. VWF is the molecule to which platelets bind during initial adhesion after blood vessel injury and is also the carrier molecule for factor VIII, protecting it from premature degradation. Thus VWD is classically characterized by both impaired platelet function (which produces prolongation of the bleeding time) and reduced factor VIIIc activity (which produces a clotting abnormality similar to, but usually less severe than, haemophilia A, with prolongation of the KPTT). In reality VWD usually presents with signs of platelet dysfunction (prolonged bleeding after minor trauma or surgical procedures, mucocutaneous bleeding, nose bleeds, menorrhagia) rather than overt features of factor VIII deficiency (haemarthrosis/muscle haematomas are rare). The platelet count is normal. Bleeding episodes are treated with DDAVP or infusions of factor VIII concentrate, depending on the severity.

3.8

a) Factor IX deficiency (also called haemophilia B or Christmas disease).

b) Factor IX assay.

The activated partial thromboplastin time (APTT) tests the 'intrinsic' clotting pathway, that is factors VIII, IX, XI and XII. Factor VIIIc is normal, which excludes haemophilia A and makes VWD unlikely. Factor XI deficiency, although prolonging the APTT, produces only clinically mild disease, and factor XII deficiency does not cause a clinically significant clotting abnormality. Therefore the most likely diagnosis is factor IX deficiency. Haemophilia A (classical haemophilia caused by factor VIII deficiency) and haemophilia B are both X-linked conditions and cannot be distinguished from each other clinically or on routine clotting tests – assays for specific clotting factor activity are required for this. Factor XIII deficiency is an autosomal recessive trait that causes a severe bleeding disorder, but the abnormality is caused by clot instability and therefore routine clotting tests are normal. It can be screened for by testing clot stability in 5M urea.

3.9

a) Disseminated intravascular coagulation (DIC) is a recognized complication of carcinoma of the prostate.

b) DIC is confirmed by measuring plasma fibrinogen (low) and fibrin degradation products (high). Renal function should also be measured since renal failure is a common complication. Other tests include a blood film to look for fragmented red blood cells (schistocytes), and LFTs (the differential diagnosis of an abnormal clotting with reduced platelet count includes liver failure).

This patient has impairment of both the intrinsic and extrinsic clotting pathways together with low platelets and anaemia.

This pattern is highly suggestive of DIC. In DIC widespread intravascular deposition of fibrin occurs, with consumption of clotting factors and platelets. Fibrin strands in the microcirculation cause fragmentation of red blood cells (schistocytes) and resultant microangiopathic haemolytic anaemia. Consumption of clotting factors and generation of FDPs result in impaired clotting with derangement of all the tests of coagulation.

3.10

a) Acute monoblastic leukaemia (M5 acute myeloid leukaemia).

Cytochemical tests can be used to determine the nature of an acute leukaemia (Table 3.1). However, it is often possible to distinguish acute myeloid (AML) from acute lymphocytic (ALL) leukaemia by morphological appearance alone: for example in AML some evidence of differentiation into granulocytes or monocytes may be seen in the blasts or their progeny (in other words the cytoplasm is granular) and the blasts often contain Auer rods, whereas in ALL the blasts show no differentiation (with the exception of B-ALL) and have very little cytoplasm.

Table 3.1 Characteristic results of cytochemical tests in acute leukaemia

Cytochemistry	ALL	AML
Sudan black	–	+
Myeloperoxidase	–	+
Periodic acid schiff (PAS)	+	– (+ in M6)
Non-specific esterase (NSE)	+	– (+ in M4; ++ in M5)

Tartrate resistant acid phosphatase is another cytochemical test that may come up in the MRCP. It is specific for, and positive in, hairy cell leukaemia (a chronic B cell leukaemia).

The type of AML is usually determined morphologically according to the FAB (French–American–British) classification shown in Box 3.3.

Box 3.3	FAB classification of AML
M1	Undifferentiated blast cells
M2	Myeloblastic
M3	Promyelocytic (associated with DIC)
M4	Myelomonocytic
M5	Monocytic (tends to infiltrate gums/perineum)
M6	Erythroleukaemia (many erythroblasts are seen*)
M7	Megakaryoblastic

*Erythroblasts may also be seen, in smaller numbers, in the other types of AML

ALL can also be divided according to an FAB classification, but is usually subdivided immunologically according to the presence or absence of specific cell surface markers.

Box 3.4 Immunological classification of ALL

Common ALL (c-ALL)
Null ALL
Pre-B ALL
B-ALL
T-ALL

3.11

a) The Paul–Bunnell test (monospot) is positive but the serology shows that the patient does not have (negative IgM), and has never had (negative IgG), EBV infection. Causes of a false positive monospot test are shown in Box 3.5.

Box 3.5 Causes of a false positive monospot test*

1. Lymphoma
2. CMV
3. Toxoplasmosis
4. Influenza
5. Hepatitis A, B, C

*All of these may also cause atypical lymphocytes on blood film

b) Lymph node biopsy since the most important condition to exclude is lymphoma.
c) CMV serology, toxoplasma serology, hepatitis serology and bone marrow aspirate and trephine biopsy are all appropriate.

The Paul–Bunnell test detects heterophile antibodies against sheep erythrocytes. These may be found in high titres in the serum of people with infectious mononucleosis but may also be found in normal people and in those suffering from serum sickness (a condition seen in the past when large doses of foreign serum, for example horse anti-diphtheria, were used for various therapeutic purposes). During the Paul–Bunnell test the patient's serum is absorbed on a suspension of guinea-pig kidney or ox red blood cells, prior to mixing with sheep erythrocytes. The heterophile antibodies of normal people or those with serum sickness are absorbed by guinea-pig kidney, but not by ox red blood cells. Their serum therefore will not cause agglutination of sheep erythrocytes after absorption on guinea-pig kidney but will be able to do so after absorption on ox red blood cells. In infectious mononucleosis the converse is true since the heterophile antibodies are absorbed by ox red blood cells, but not by guinea-pig kidney. Modern slide screening kits (monospot test) use formalized horse red cells, which are more sensitive, instead of sheep erythrocytes.

3.12

a) Aplastic crisis caused by parvovirus (B19 usually) infection.

The child has suddenly become severely anaemic. The low reticulocyte count indicates that this is the result of bone marrow aplasia rather than haemolysis, in which one would expect to see a high reticulocyte count. Infection with parvovirus B19 causes a short period of suppression of bone marrow erythropoiesis. In normal people this is not clinically significant, but in those with reduced red cell lifespan (for example sickle-cell disease, thalassaemias, hereditary spherocytosis or pyruvate kinase deficiency), aplastic crisis may occur during which there is rapid worsening of the anaemia. Aplastic crisis can also occur because of folate deficiency and folate supplementation is therefore essential in these conditions.

3.13

a) The presence of a large number of blasts in the peripheral blood indicates that this man has acute leukaemia and the presence of disseminated intravascular coagulation suggests that promyelocytic (M3) acute myeloid leukaemia is the correct diagnosis.

b) Disseminated intravascular coagulation is indicated by the presence of deranged clotting with a low fibrinogen, thrombocytopenia and the presence of schistocytes (fragmented red cells) on the blood film. DIC is extremely common in this form of leukaemia.

c) Bone marrow aspirate and trephine biopsy, fibrin degradation products (FDPs), and cytochemical tests to determine the nature of the blast cells are all indicated. If stuck for an answer then HLA typing for possible bone marrow transplantation is also worth mentioning.

3.14

a) Immune thrombocytopenic purpura (ITP).

b) Appropriate tests are anti-platelet autoantibodies and bone marrow aspirate and trephine biopsy (to exclude acute leukaemia). In autoimmune (idiopathic) thrombocytopenic purpura the bone marrow will show hyperplasia of the megakaryocytes in response to peripheral destruction of platelets caused by platelet autoantibodies.

Immune thrombocytopenic purpura is the commonest cause of thrombocytopenia without anaemia or neutropenia. The acute form of ITP is most common in children and in 75% of cases follows vaccination or viral infection such as measles, chicken pox or infectious mononucleosis. It usually resolves spontaneously but may become chronic in 5–10% of cases. The chronic form is more common in adults, especially women aged 15–50 years, and is usually idiopathic although it may occur in association with other diseases (for example SLE, HIV infection, CLL, Hodgkin's disease or autoimmune haemolytic anaemia) in which case it is called Evans syndrome. Unlike the acute childhood form, chronic ITP rarely resolves spontaneously. Treatment includes high-dose corticosteroids (which produce remission in 80%) progressing to splenectomy and immunosuppressive drugs such as cyclophosphamide or azathioprine in those that do not respond to steroids. Life-threatening thrombocytopenia can be partially corrected with immunoglobulin infusions, which produce a rapid rise in the platelet count. Anabolic steroids such as danazol may be useful for restoring the platelet count in refractory cases.

3.15

a) Thrombotic thrombocytopenic purpura (Moschkovitz syndrome).

TTP is a condition that mainly affects young adults and is characterized by severe thrombocytopenia, microangiopathic haemolytic anaemia, confluent purpura and widespread ischaemic organ damage (caused by deposition of platelet microthrombi), which results in fluctuating neurological signs and renal failure. Unlike DIC, however, the clotting is normal. Plasma exchange and infusions of fresh frozen plasma are the mainstay of treatment but aspirin, azathioprine and cyclophosphamide may also be used.

The exact pathogenesis is unknown but it may occur in association with SLE and other connective tissue disorders, pregnancy (usually antepartum and tends to recur in subsequent pregnancies) and carcinoma or lymphoma.

The haemolytic–uraemic syndrome (HUS; see Q 3.17) is similar but mainly (though not exclusively) affects children. Organ damage is limited to the kidneys and neurological symptoms and signs are therefore classically not a feature (although this is not strictly speaking true). It is becoming increasingly recognized that HUS and TTP have similar causes (Box 3.6) and are part of the same spectrum of disease.

Box 3.6 Causes of a microangiopathic haemolytic anaemia (TTP or HUS)

1. Infection
    Verocytotoxin-producing strains of *E. coli*
    Shigella
    HIV

2. Connective tissue disorders
    SLE
    Scleroderma crisis

3. Malignant hypertension
4. Malignancy (mainly adenocarcinomas)
5. Pregnancy   usually antepartum (< 6 months) and tends to recur with subsequent pregnancies
6. Drugs   Ticlopidine, oral contraceptive pill, 5-FU, cyclosporin, mitomycin-C
7. Post-transplantation

3.16

a) Haemolytic anaemia secondary to dapsone treatment. Dapsone causes oxidative damage to erythrocytes, which can result in intravascular haemolysis (reflected by the presence of fragmented red cells [schistocytes] on the blood film). Reticulocytosis is a physiological response to loss of red cells from whatever cause (haemolysis or blood loss).

b) Heinz bodies, which consist of oxidized, denatured haemoglobin and are a sign of oxidative stress. These are mainly seen in splenectomized patients, but gluten-sensitive enteropathy may be associated with hyposplenism.

c) Dermatitis herpetiformis may be associated with a gluten-sensitive enteropathy, thus iron and/or folate deficiency may also be contributing to the anaemia. Folate deficiency may also be a consequence of increased folate requirement caused by haemolysis.

Sulphonamides are the other main class of drug that may be associated with a Heinz body haemolytic anaemia in normal individuals. In contrast, many drugs that impose oxidative stress on the red cell may produce this type of anaemia in those with G6PD deficiency (see answer to Q 3.18).

3.17

a) Haemolytic–uraemic syndrome (HUS) or disseminated intravascular coagulation (DIC).

b) Investigations should include: clotting screen (normal in HUS), fibrin degradation products (FDPs) and fibrinogen. All of these indices are normal in HUS, whereas in DIC clotting is deranged, FDPs are elevated and fibrinogen is reduced.

c) Further investigation should include: direct Coombs' test (to exclude autoimmune haemolytic anaemia); arterial blood gases to look for acidosis; and renal ultrasound (to exclude an obstructive cause for renal failure, or pre-existing chronic renal failure). Other useful investigations include: reticulocyte count, blood film (to look for schistocytes) and stool culture.

d) Acidosis may result in hyperventilation (respiratory compensation).

Although HUS usually occurs in children, it can also occur in adults, therefore do not be fooled by the patient's age. HUS is characterized by microangiopathic haemolysis, thrombocytopenia and acute renal failure. Clinically it is similar to TTP but neurological symptoms/signs are not a feature. The pathogenesis is unknown but it often occurs following an acute febrile illness, especially those caused by verocytotoxin producing strains of *E. coli* (VTEC) or respiratory tract infections. Deposition of fibrin and platelet microthrombi, particularly in the kidneys, results in renal failure, platelet consumption and red cell fragmentation. Clotting studies FDPs and fibrinogen are normal, however, unlike in DIC (see also answer to Q 3.9).

3.18

a) Glucose 6 phosphate dehydrogenase deficiency (G6PD deficiency).

b) Other conditions in which there is chronic haemolysis include: hereditary spherocytosis or elliptocytosis, and pyruvate kinase deficiency.

c) Investigations should be aimed at distinguishing between the differential diagnoses. Appropriate investigations include:

- Red cell G6PD assay. This should not be performed until at least six weeks after the acute haemolytic episode since the young red blood cells released in response to haemolysis have normal enzyme activity.
- Blood film. 'Bite' and 'blister' cells (cells which have had Heinz bodies removed by the spleen) or Heinz bodies (these consist of oxidized, denatured haemoglobin and are a sign of oxidative stress) may be seen in a haemolytic crisis in G6PD deficiency, whereas spherocytes suggest hereditary spherocytosis.
- Osmotic fragility studies. Osmotic fragility of the red cells is increased in hereditary spherocytosis. Autohaemolysis (the degree of haemolysis when the cells are incubated in their own serum for 24 h) is also increased, but is corrected by addition of glucose.

d) Some anti-malarial tablets cause oxidative stress and may result in a haemolytic crisis (Box 3.7). It is therefore important for the family to seek specialist advice about safe and effective malaria prophylaxis prior to travelling to Africa.

Box 3.7 Commonly used drugs that may cause haemolysis in G6PD deficiency

1. Anti-malarials
    Chloroquine
    Quinidine
    Quinine
    Primaquine
    Pentaquine
    Pamaquine

2. Sulphonamides (including cotrimoxazole)

3. Quinolones
    Ciprofloxacin
    Ofloxacin
    Nalidixic acid

4. Nitrofurantoin

5. Dapsone

6. Probenecid

7. Methylene blue

Reticulocytosis and the presence of elevated unconjugated bilirubin (there is no bilirubin in the urine despite elevated plasma total bilirubin levels) suggest haemolysis. The Hb is normal, indicating that the haemolysis is currently compensated by increased bone marrow cell turnover. However, this child has had periods during which he is clinically jaundiced in the past, which implies that the degree of haemolysis has worsened on occasions. Thus the clinical picture is one of chronic low level haemolysis with intermittent exacerbations. This suggests G6PD deficiency; this is an X-linked disorder and therefore only males are affected. The enzyme is necessary for production of NADPH via the pentose monophosphate shunt pathway and NADPH is required to keep glutathione in its reduced state. Reduced glutathione protects the red cell membrane and haemoglobin from oxidative damage. Thus during oxidative stress (which can be caused by infection, acute illness, fava or broad beans, and many drugs) acute haemolysis occurs in patients with G6PD deficiency. Since the bone marrow can compensate for low level chronic haemolysis the haemoglobin is normal between attacks. This is in contrast to hereditary sphero/eliptocytosis or pyruvate kinase deficiency where the patient is anaemic, to varying degrees, all of the time.

3.19

a) Ring sideroblasts.

Although the blood film shows microspherocytes, the MCV is macrocytic indicating that the film is actually dimorphic. Causes of a dimorphic blood film include, amongst other things, secondary acquired sideroblastic anaemia which may be caused by both alcoholism (the patient is a publican) and isoniazid therapy (which this patient is probably taking as part of his anti-tuberculous chemotherapy). Pyrazinamide, which may be used in the treatment of TB, can also cause sideroblastic anaemia. In sideroblastic anaemia, a defect in haem synthesis results in the presence of numerous iron granules arranged in a ring around the nucleus, instead of the few randomly distributed iron granules that are normally seen when erythroblasts are stained for iron. Repeated transfusions are usually required for severe cases, but some patients may respond to pyridoxine supplements.

3.20

a) Porphyria cutanea tarda.

b) Urinary uroporphyrin is elevated in this condition. Liver biopsy and staining for iron should also be performed.

c) Venesection to a haemoglobin concentration of less than 12 g/dl may induce remission. Chloroquine can be used to promote urinary porphyrin excretion.

Porphyria cutanea tarda is the commonest form of porphyria. It is usually only expressed in the presence of hepatic damage from some other cause, particularly alcohol and/or haemochromatosis. Although in this patient the elevated gamma GT and low platelet count suggest alcoholism, liver biopsy and staining for iron should be performed to exclude haemochromatosis. Reduced serum iron binding capacity together with increased serum iron and ferritin are often seen in porphyria cutanea tarda (see also answer to Q 3.21).

3.21

a) Acute intermittent porphyria. Sulphonamides are one of the many classes of drug that can cause attacks of acute porphyria, and cotrimoxazole consists of trimethoprim together with the sulphonamide, sulphamethoxazole.

b) Appropriate investigations are:
- Urinary porphobilinogen (PBG) and delta aminolaevulinic acid (δALA), which are elevated in acute attacks of acute intermittent porphyria.
- Assay of red cell PBG deaminase (reduced) and δALA synthetase (increased) gives the definitive diagnosis.
- Plasma:urine osmolality ratio to demonstrate SIADH, which is associated with acute intermittent porphyria and may be the cause of this patient's low sodium.

c) Stop the cotrimoxazole. The other family members should be screened by assay of their red cell PBG deaminase and ALA synthetase activity.

HAEMATOLOGY

THE PORPHYRIAS

These are a group of inherited disorders (mainly autosomal dominant) which result from deficiency of one of the enzymes of the haem synthetic pathway.

For the purposes of the MRCP exam, there are basically two phenotypes: the acute porphyrias, of which acute intermittent porphyria is the prime example; and the cutaneous porphyrias, of which porphyria cutanea tarda is the most common. In reality, however, things are not quite this simple, and whereas the non-acute porphyrias show only cutaneous symptoms, all of the acute porphyrias, with the exception of acute intermittent porphyria, may have cutaneous involvement as well.

In the acute porphyrias, δALA and PBG accumulate, and are excreted in increased quantities in the urine. The levels of δALA and PBG correlate well with the symptoms, which are mainly neurological in origin. Symptoms include: abdominal pain, vomiting and constipation (90%); peripheral neuropathies (70%; mainly motor); hypertension and tachycardia caused by autonomic neuropathy (70%); and neuropsychiatric disturbance (50%) such as seizures, depression or frank psychosis. In the exam always consider acute intermittent porphyria in the differential diagnosis of the person who presents with both abdominal and neurological symptoms, or neurological symptoms with hypertension and a tachycardia. Between acute attacks (the latent phase) urinary δALA and PBG excretion is normal, and for this reason urine testing is not sufficient as a screening tool; the red cell enzymes have to be directly assayed for this purpose.

In the purely cutaneous forms of porphyria (the non-acute forms) δALA and PBG do not accumulate. However, accumulation of porphyrins in the upper epidermal layer of the skin causes a photosensitive rash with subepidermal blisters.

3.22

a) Lead poisoning.

b) Acute porphyria (abdominal pain with neurological symptoms may be the presenting feature of acute intermittent porphyria).

c) Appropriate investigations include: urinary coproporphyrin levels (raised in lead poisoning); X-ray of long bones (wrist and knee) for dense metaphyseal bands (lead lines); and plasma lead levels (but these may be variable).

Lead poisoning inhibits several of the enzymes involved in haem synthesis and eventually causes anaemia. In addition it interferes with the breakdown of RNA by inhibiting the enzyme pyrimidine 5′ nucleotidase. This causes accumulation of denatured RNA in red cells, which gives the appearance of basophilic stippling on ordinary (Romanowski) staining. Lead also binds to bones and teeth causing bluish 'lead lines'. Symptoms consist of anorexia, nausea, vomiting, constipation, severe abdominal pain (which may resemble the 'acute abdomen'), peripheral motor neuropathies (for example wrist or foot drop) and lead encephalopathy which may cause seizures. Although the symptoms may resemble those of acute intermittent porphyria, urinary PBG excretion is not usually elevated. Urinary δALA and coproporphyrin levels are, however, elevated in lead poisoning and can be used, in conjunction with the absence of PBG, as a diagnostic test. Lead poisoning can be actively treated with chelating agents such as calcium EDTA, D-penicillamine or dimercaprol.

4 RENAL MEDICINE

4.1

See also questions 5.1, 5.3 and 5.5

a) Membranous glomerulonephritis (membranous nephropathy).

b) The causes of membranous glomerulonephritis are shown in Box 4.1.

Box 4.1 Causes of membranous glomerulonephritis
1. Connective tissue diseases e.g. rheumatoid arthritis, SLE
2. Malignancy (underlying cause in 10% of cases)
   Carcinoma of bronchus, colon, stomach, prostate or breast
   Hodgkin's or non-Hodgkin's lymphoma
3. Infections: hepatitis B, syphilis, filariasis, leprosy, malaria
4. Drugs: gold, penicillamine, captopril

---

c) Renal vein thrombosis.

This patient has nephrotic syndrome (proteinuria > 5 g/24 h, hypoalbuminaemia and generalized oedema ± hypercholesterolaemia). The causes of nephrotic syndrome are shown in Box 4.2, but by far the commonest causes are the glomeronephritides, particularly minimal change and membranous GN. The electron microscopy appearance of the renal biopsy is characteristic of membranous GN and immunofluorescence would show granular deposits of IgG and C3 on the subepithelial surface of the glomerular basement membrane. In the case of minimal change GN the electron micrograph would show fusion of the podocyte foot processes and there would be no immune complexes seen on electron microscopy. Patients with nephrotic syndrome have a hypercoagulable state because of a number of alterations in both prothrombotic and anti-thrombotic proteins and are therefore at risk of both arterial and venous thromboses. Renal vein thrombosis should always be suspected if there is a sudden and unexplained deterioration in renal function. It is often asymptomatic but may be associated with loin pain and/or haematuria. Renal vein thrombosis occurs in 10–20% of those with nephrotic syndrome and in 30% of those with membranous glomerulonephritis. The diagnosis is confirmed by renal venogram or, more recently, by CT scan of the renal veins. Treatment is with intravenous heparin but anti-thrombin-3 may need to be given before the heparin is effective (because of renal loss). Other complications of nephrotic syndrome include hypercholesterolaemia (↑LDL ± ↑VLDL), susceptibility to infections (loss of immunoglobulins in the urine) and reduced binding proteins (renal loss).

Box 4.2 Causes of nephrotic syndrome

Glomerulonephritis
Minimal change GN
Membranous GN
Focal segmental glomerulosclerosis
Membranoproliferative GN

Systemic diseases
Diabetes mellitus (diabetic nephrosclerosis)
Connective tissue diseases e.g. SLE
Small vessel vasculitides
Amyloidosis

Infections
Bacterial: Post-streptococcal, syphilis, endocarditis, shunt nephritis
Viral: HBV, HCV, HIV, EBV, CMV
Parasitic: Malaria, toxoplasmosis, filariasis, schistosomiasis

Tumour-associated
Hodgkin's (associated with minimal change or membranous GN)
Solid tumours (associated with membranous GN)

Drugs
Gold and other heavy metals, penicillamine, captopril, NSAIDs, lithium

Other
Allergens, venoms, immunizations
Pregnancy (including pre-eclampsia)
Unilateral renal artery stenosis
Reflux nephropathy
Sickle-cell disease
Alport syndrome
Fabry's disease
Familial

4.2

a) Pre-renal failure caused by inadequate fluid replacement.

b) Urine microscopy and culture (to screen for urinary infection, and rare causes of renal failure such as interstitial nephritis, vasculitis and glomerulonephritis) and renal ultrasound (to exclude acute obstruction caused for instance by clot retention) are indicated. In general, these tests should always be performed in patients with acute renal failure.

This patient may have a pre-renal, renal or post-renal cause for his renal failure. The latter is less likely since his catheter is draining, albeit small volumes, and the pre-op renal function was normal, making a chronic obstructive lesion unlikely. A renal ultrasound is still required to exclude this possibility though. Given the recent history of hypovolaemia the two most likely causes are pre-renal failure caused by inadequate fluid replacement, or acute tubular necrosis secondary to the hypotensive episode. The biochemical features of each of these is shown in Table 4.1. This patient is producing small volumes of concentrated urine containing little sodium (evidence of activation of the renin-aldosterone system secondary to reduced renal blood flow), which suggests pre-renal failure.

Table 4.1 Classical urinary indices of acute tubular necrosis vs. pre-renal failure

	Pre-renal	Acute tubular necrosis
Urinary osmolarity (mosm/L)	> 500	< 350
Urinary sodium (mmol/L)	< 20	> 20
Urinary/plasma urea ratio	> 8	< 3
Urinary/plasma creatinine ratio	> 40	< 20
Fractional sodium excretion	< 1	> 1

*Intermediate values are common and values will be affected by diuretics or pre-existing renal disease

4.3

a) IgA nephropathy (otherwise known as Burger's disease or mesangioproliferative glomerulonephritis).

b) Renal biopsy.

c) Light microscopy will show a mesangioproliferative (focal proliferative) glomerular nephritis. Immunofluorescence is diagnostic, showing globular mesangial deposits of IgA and C3.

This patient has developed nephritis (renal impairment with haematuria and proteinuria) following an acute upper respiratory tract infection. The causes of this clinical scenario are IgA nephropathy, post-streptococcal (post-infectious) glomerulonephritis or acute interstitial nephritis associated with infectious mononucleosis. The latter condition is rare, and post-streptococcal glomerulonephritis classically occurs 2–3 weeks after the infection rather than within the first few days as in this case.

IgA nephropathy is the commonest form of glomerulonephritis worldwide. It classically presents with recurrent episodes of acute nephritis, associated with myalgia, malaise and loin pain, beginning within 24–48 hours of an URTI, typically pharyngitis. However, about one-third of cases present with asymptomatic, persistent microscopic haematuria +/or proteinuria. IgA nephropathy may also occur as part of Henoch–Schönlein purpura. There are no serological markers for this condition (although IgA may be elevated) and diagnosis is confirmed by renal biopsy – the immunofluorescence pattern is characteristic, although mesangial IgA deposits may also occur in lupus nephritis, cirrhosis, coeliac disease and HIV nephropathy. Complement levels are normal.

Post-infectious glomerulonephritis classically presents with acute nephritis (urine is said to be 'smoky' in appearance rather than the frank haematuria seen with IgA nephropathy) 2–3 weeks after an URTI due to group A β haemolytic streptococcus. Oliguria, fluid retention (oedema) and hypertension are common. Other presentations include asymptomatic microscopic haematuria +/or proteinuria and the nephrotic syndrome. Serum C3 is typically reduced and the ASOT is positive. Renal biopsy is not usually necessary. In most cases the renal impairment resolves within a few weeks but haematuria and proteinuria may persist for many months.

4.4

a) Membranoproliferative (mesangiocapillary) glomerulonephritis type II.

b) Membranoproliferative glomerulonephritis type I, lupus nephritis or essential mixed cryoglobulinaemia.

c) Autoantibody screen (including ANA, anti-dsDNA and ANCA), cryoglobulins and renal biopsy with immunofluorescence staining are indicated.

d) C3 nephritic factor.

Red cell casts in the centrifuged urinary sediment are indicative of either glomerulonephritis, vasculitis or interstitial nephritis (red cell casts are only occasionally found in interstitial nephritis). However, reduced serum complement is more characteristic of certain types of GN (Box 4.3). There is no history of recent infection, no clinical evidence of infective endocarditis and this patient does not have a ventriculoatrial shunt. Thus membranoproliferative GN types I and II, lupus nephritis and essential mixed cryoglobulinaemia remain as the differential diagnoses that are suggested by the data. (**NB**: The GN seen in essential mixed cryoglobulinaemia is actually membranoproliferative GN type I; however, membranoproliferative GN also occurs in the absence of cryoglobulinaemia so the two conditions have been listed separately.) The presence of partial lipodystrophy and normal C4 favours membranoproliferative GN type II (although in reality this is exceedingly rare).

Differentiation between the possible diagnoses ultimately requires renal biopsy. In addition to looking for the characteristic histological features, immunofluorescence of the biopsy specimen should also be performed. It characteristically shows glomerular and extraglomerular deposits of IgG, IgM and complement in lupus nephritis; granular subendothelial deposits of IgG and C3 in membranoproliferative GN type I (and mixed cryoglobulinaemia), and mesangial deposits of C3 only in membranoproliferative GN type II.

Membranoproliferative GN presents with either nephrotic syndrome (one-third), acute nephritis (one-third) or asymptomatic haematuria and/or proteinuria (one-third). Type I may be associated with HCV infection (in which case essential mixed cryoglobulinaemia is the underlying disease: see answer to Q 5.2), although the majority of cases are idiopathic. Type 2 may be associated with partial lipodystrophy and/or the presence of C3 nephritic factor. This is an antibody (IgG) directed against C3bBb of the alternative complement pathway causing continuous activation of this pathway and, consequently, reduced C3. Electron microscopy shows subendothelial electron dense deposits in type I and subepithelial electron dense deposits in type II.

RENAL MEDICINE

> **Box 4.3 Glomerulonephritis associated with low C3**
>
> *C1 and C4 usually low also*
>   Lupus nephritis
>   Bacterial endocarditis
>   Shunt nephritis
>   Essential cryoglobulinaemia
>   Membranoproliferative (mesangiocapillary) glomerulonephritis type I
>
> *C1 and C4 usually normal*
>   Membranoproliferative (mesangiocapillary) glomerulonephritis type II
>   Post-infectious glomerulonephritis
>
> All of the above may also occur with normal complement levels

4.5

a) Lupus nephritis.

b) Renal biopsy, serum paraproteins and urinary Bence-Jones protein, and anti-nuclear antibody (found in 95% of cases of SLE but lacks specificity) are all indicated. Serum complement C3 and C4 (reduced in active lupus), anti-dsDNA antibody (specific for SLE but only found in 50% of cases; levels correlate with disease activity in lupus nephritis) and biopsy of normal skin (linear band of IgG and C3 at dermoepidermal junction in SLE) may also be useful. Twenty-four hour urine protein estimation, U + E and creatinine clearance are also indicated but these would not lead to a diagnosis.

This patient has proteinuria with a high ESR, positive VDRL and thrombocytopenia. The proteinuria and high ESR are not caused by urinary infection (urine culture negative) and diabetic nephropathy is an unlikely cause, despite the presence of glycosuria, since fasting blood glucose is normal (lupus nephritis is often associated with a degree of tubular dysfunction so a low renal threshold for glucose is the cause of the glycosuria in this case). This leaves glomerulonephritis and multiple myeloma as the main possibilities. Syphilis can be associated with membranous glomerulonephritis and, although the VDRL is positive, the *Treponema pallidum* haemagglutination test (TPHA), which is more specific than VDRL, is negative, excluding syphilis. False positive tests for VDRL occur in lupus because of the presence of anti-phospholipid antibodies. CRP is characteristically normal (or only marginally elevated) in SLE despite elevation of other measures of inflammation such as ESR. Finally, thrombocytopenia (and other 'penias) are extremely common in active lupus.

Several drugs are associated with an SLE-like syndrome, but drug-induced SLE characteristically does not involve the kidney (or the CNS).

Box 4.4 Drugs associated with drug-induced SLE

1. Hydralazine
2. Isoniazid
3. Phenytoin
4. Chlorpromazine
5. Methyldopa
6. Procainamide
7. Ethosuxamide

4.6

a) Right renal artery stenosis.

b) A dense but delayed nephrogram will be seen on the intravenous pyelogram.

c) Renal angiography or renal magnetic resonance angiography is the gold standard and should be performed to confirm the diagnosis and determine whether stenosis is caused by atheromatous disease (stenosis located at or near the junction of the renal artery and the aorta; aorta also atheromatous; often evidence of atheromatous disease elsewhere) or fibrous dysplasia (alternating stenosis and dilatation, which is characteristically in the distal two-thirds of the renal artery and produces a 'string of beads' appearance; aorta normal).

In renal artery stenosis glomerular filtration pressure, in the face of reduced renal blood flow, is maintained by angiotensin II-mediated vasoconstriction of the efferent arteriole. When captopril is given this vasoconstriction is lost and renal function consequently falls. Thus in the post-captopril renogram the right kidney is seen to contribute considerably less to the overall renal function.

Other tests that may come up in the MRCP are:

- *Renal vein renin ratio:* blood samples are taken from each renal vein and assayed for renin. A ratio of > 1.6 is strongly suggestive of renal artery stenosis, with the highest renin level being on the side of the stenosis.
- *Captopril challenge test:* plasma renin activity is measured before and 60 min after captopril. An exaggerated increase is seen in renal artery stenosis.

FLUID BALANCE

The water deprivation test

This involves depriving the subject of all fluids for 8 h while measuring weight and taking blood and urine samples for osmolality measurements every 2 h. The patient is then given 2 μg of the ADH analogue desmopressin (DDAVP) intramuscularly and urine samples are collected over the next 12–16 h. The test should be stopped if there is weight loss of > 5% or when the urine osmolality has risen to > 750 mOsm/kg. Interpretation of the results is outlined in Table 4.2.

Table 4.2 Expected values for urine osmolality during water deprivation test (mOsm/kg)

	Following water deprivation	Following DDAVP
Normal*	> 750	no further rise
Complete cranial diabetes insipidus	< 300	rises by > 50%
Partial cranial diabetes insipidus	300–750 (partial concentration)	rises by > 10%
Nephrogenic diabetes insipidus	< 300	no further rise
Psychogenic polydipsia	300–750 (partial concentration)	no further rise because of medullary washout

*Normal range for plasma osmolality = 278–305 mOsm/kg
Normal range of urine osmolality = 60–1500 mOsm/kg.

4.7

a) Psychogenic polydipsia.

b) Water deprivation test.

This patient is passing large volumes of dilute urine yet still has a low plasma osmolality. If she had diabetes insipidus one would expect her plasma osmolality to be high normal (or normal).

4.8

a) Cranial diabetes insipidus.

The urine osmolality is low and does not increase much during fluid deprivation showing that diabetes insipidus is present. But there is a significant rise after DDAVP indicating that the kidney is responsive to vasopressin. Deficient central production/excretion of vasopressin must therefore be present: that is, cranial diabetes insipidus.

b) Histiocytosis X.

Histiocytosis X is a rare malignant condition characterized by infiltration of monoclonal Langerhans-like cells and eosinophils, producing destructive lytic lesions. It can affect many different tissues including bone, liver, spleen, brain and skin. It can also be associated with pulmonary fibrosis producing 'honeycomb lung'. If it involves the hypothalamus or pituitary it can cause cranial diabetes insipidus.

Box 4.5 Causes of cranial diabetes insipidus	
1. Trauma e.g.	Head injury
	Surgery
	CVA
	Sheehan syndrome
	DXT
2. Infiltration by	
a) Tumours e.g.	Craniopharyngioma
	Pituitary adenomas
	Hypothalamic tumours
	Lymphoma/leukaemia
	Histiocytosis X
	Metastases
b) Sarcoidosis	
3. Infection e.g.	TB
	Basal meningitis (syphilis)
	Cerebral abscess
4. Autoimmune e.g.	SLE
5. Idiopathic	

RENAL MEDICINE

4.9

a) Nephrogenic diabetes insipidus.

The urine osmolality increases very little during water deprivation, and does not change significantly even after DDAVP indicating that the renal tubules are not responsive to vasopressin, and thus nephrogenic diabetes insipidus is indicated.

b) Glibenclamide is a sulphonylurea that can cause nephrogenic diabetes insipidus. A previous episode of pyelonephritis could also be responsible for this condition.

Box 4.6 Causes of nephrogenic diabetes insipidus	
1. Renal damage e.g.	Hydronephrosis Pyelonephritis Sickle cell disease
2. Associated with renal tubular acidosis	
3. Metabolic e.g.	Hypokalaemia Hypercalcaemia
4. Drugs e.g.	Lithium Amphotericin Glibenclamide Demeclocycline and outdated tetracyclines

4.10

a) Psychogenic polydipsia.

The renal tubules do have some concentrating ability as shown by the rise in the urine osmolality from 300 to 500 during water deprivation. However the high urine output associated with psychogenic polydipsia washes out urea from the renal medulla thus reducing the ability of the kidneys to concentrate urine fully. Characteristically there is no further concentration of the urine when DDAVP is given. Partial cranial or partial nephrogenic diabetes insipidus (DI) may cause diagnostic confusion since in these conditions the kidneys are also able to partially concentrate the urine during water deprivation. However, in partial cranial DI there will be further concentration of the urine after DDAVP is given. Partial nephrogenic DI can be differentiated by simultaneous measurement of plasma ADH, which will be inappropriately high with respect to the low urine osmolality in nephrogenic DI.

4.11

a) Syndrome of inappropriate ADH secretion (SIADH).
b) *Mycoplasma pneumoniae* chest infection.

Box 4.7 Causes of SIADH	
1. Pulmonary lesions e.g.	TB Pneumonia (especially *Mycoplasma*) Abscess Aspergillus IPPV
2. CNS lesions e.g.	Meningoencephalitis Abscess Stroke Subarachnoid haemorrhage Subdural haematoma Head injury Vasculitis (e.g. SLE) Guillain–Barré syndrome
3. Malignancy e.g.	Small cell lung Pancreas Duodenum Urothelial Prostate Lymphoma/leukaemia Adrenal Thymus
4. Metabolic e.g.	Alcohol withdrawal Acute intermittent porphyria Hypothyroidism
5. Drugs e.g.	Opiates Chlorpropamide Antipsychotics (e.g. chlorpromazine) Thiazides Carbamazepine Barbiturates Bromocriptine Rifampicin Cytotoxics (e.g. vincristine, cyclophosphamide)

The plasma osmolality is calculated from the following equation:

$$\text{Plasma osmolality (mOsm/kg)} = 2 \times ([Na^+] + [K^+]) + [\text{urea}] + [\text{glucose}]$$

In this case the value is 260 mOsm/kg. Since the urine osmolality is 580 mOsm/kg, the urine:plasma osmolality ratio is > 2:1, which meets the diagnostic criterion for SIADH. SIADH is an important cause of hyponatraemia and can be caused by all types of pulmonary infection but is particularly associated with *Mycoplasma pneumoniae* infections.

4.12

a) Chronic alcoholism.

The calculated plasma osmolality is 285 mOsm/kg yet the measured plasma osmolality is 328 mOsm/kg. The difference (in this case 43 mOsm/kg) is called the 'osmolar gap' and is caused by the presence of an osmotically active substance not normally found in the blood in sufficient quantities to be included in the calculation of osmolality. It is however detected in the direct assay of plasma osmolality, hence the discrepancy. Such substances include ketones, ethanol, methanol and ethylene glycol. Renal failure can also result in an increased osmolar gap through retention of various organic and inorganic molecules. This patient does not have ketoacidosis (glucose normal) and is not in renal failure. Therefore the most likely cause of the elevated osmolar gap is alcohol and the low urea suggests chronic alcohol abuse.

ACID-BASE BALANCE

Table 4.3 Acids within the body

Acid	Source
1. $CO_2 \Leftrightarrow H^+ + HCO_3$	Tissue respiration

2. Organic acids:
    Lactate
    FFAs
    Ketones: [hydroxybutyrate, acetoacetic acid]
	Products of metabolism

3. Fixed acids: [sulphuric, phosphoric]	Foods

Disturbances of acid-base balance

These may be recognized as shown in Table 4.4.

Table 4.4 Diagnostic features of acid-base disturbances

Type of acid-base disturbance	Principal abnormality	Compensatory change
Metabolic acidosis	↓ HCO_3^-	↓ $paCO_2$
Respiratory acidosis	↑ $paCO_2$	↑ HCO_3^-
Metabolic alkalosis	↑ HCO_3^-	↑ $paCO_2$ (slight)
Respiratory alkalosis	↓ $paCO_2$	↓ HCO_3^-

Anion gap

This is calculated by subtracting the sum of the plasma concentrations of the main anions from that of the main cations. It represents the unestimated anions, which consist of negatively charged proteins, phosphate and organic acids. The normal value of the anion gap is 10–18 mmol/L.

$$(Na^+ + K^+) - (HCO_3^- + Cl^-) \cong 10\text{–}18 \, mmol/L$$
$\quad\quad$ cations $\quad\quad\quad$ main anions $\quad\quad\quad$ anion gap

High anion gap metabolic acidosis

Caused by retention of fixed or organic acids (↑ production / ↓ excretion). See Box 4.8.

Box 4.8 Causes of high anion gap metabolic acidosis

1. Uraemia

2. Ketoacidosis e.g.   Diabetes
                                    Starvation
                                    Alcohol

3. Lactic acidosis e.g.   Shock
                                    Hypoxia
                                    Bigunides
                                    Liver failure
                                    Trauma

4. Ingestion of acids e.g.   Salicylates
                                       Ethylene glycol

Normal anion gap (hyperchloraemic) metabolic acidosis

Chloride ions (Cl^-) are retained to balance the charge of the bicarbonate ions (HCO_3^-) which are lost. The causes are shown in Box 4.9.

RENAL MEDICINE

> **Box 4.9 Causes of normal anion gap (hyperchloraemic) metabolic acidosis**
>
> 1. Loss of HCO_3^-
>   a) From the gut e.g.
>   Diarrhoea
>   Pancreatic fistula
>   Ureterosigmoidostomy
>   b) From the kidney e.g.:
>   Renal tubular acidosis
>   Carbonic anhydrase inhibitors
> 2. Rarely caused by ingestion of acid e.g.
> H^+ as NH_4Cl
>   IV feeds with excess cationic amino acids

Loss of anion gap

Box 4.10 lists the causes of anion gap loss.

> **Box 4.10 Causes of loss of anion gap**
>
> 1. Paraproteinaemia
>   (High positive charge on paraproteins → retention of Cl^-)
> 2. Hypoalbuminaemia
>   (Loss of negative charge has same effect as high positive charge)
> 3. Hypermagnesaemia
>   (Mg^{++} has high positive charge)
> 4. Bromide intake

4.13

a) High anion gap metabolic acidosis.

b) Lactic acidosis secondary to poor tissue perfusion resulting from hypothermia and hypotension.

c) Serum lactate.

This patient has a low bicarbonate together with low $paCO_2$. Reference to Table 4.4 in the introductory notes to this section reveals that this can be caused by metabolic acidosis or respiratory alkalosis. However, in the case of an alkalosis one would expect the potassium to be low, so metabolic acidosis is the most likely cause. You have been given enough information to calculate the anion gap and should therefore do so. Using the equation in the introductory notes above, this is calculated to be 46.8, which is high. The causes of a high anion gap metabolic acidosis are shown in Box 4.8.

4.14

a) Compensated respiratory acidosis.

The $paCO_2$ is high with a pH towards the lower end of the normal range suggesting that acidosis is the primary abnormality. Compensation has occurred by retention of bicarbonate and this has brought the pH back into the normal range.

4.15

a) Mixed respiratory and metabolic acidosis.

b) Pneumonia has caused a respiratory acidosis and has also precipitated diabetic ketoacidosis.

This patient is clearly acidotic. A pure metabolic acidosis would cause low bicarbonate with a low $paCO_2$ (caused by attempted respiratory compensation). Conversely a pure respiratory acidosis would cause a high $paCO_2$ with low bicarbonate (through attempted renal compensation). The combined metabolic and respiratory acidosis produces a high $paCO_2$ with low bicarbonate since ventilatory impairment prevents any respiratory compensation for the metabolic component of the acidosis.

4.16

a) Renal tubular acidosis type 1 (distal).

b) Sjögren syndrome; hypergammaglobulinaemia; primary biliary cirrhosis (see Box 4.11 for other causes).

c) The chloride will be high since renal tubular acidosis is associated with a normal anion gap (i.e. hyperchloraemic) metabolic acidosis.

K^+ is normally elevated in acidosis since H^+ is preferentially excreted in the distal tubule under these conditions. The combination of acidosis and low K^+ is strongly suggestive of renal tubular acidosis. Low serum calcium together with renal calculi make the distal form most likely. Low phosphate is caused by secondary hyperparathyroidism.

In type 1 renal tubular acidosis (distal tubule) the distal tubular cells are abnormally permeable to H^+, which results in re-entry of H^+ into the tubular cells. High intracellular H^+ concentration inhibits carbonic anhydrase and hence $HCO3^-$ production. Diagnosis is from a first morning urine (pH < 5.3 excludes distal RTA) or, more formally, by a NH_4Cl acid-load test (failure to acidify urine when given acid load confirms diagnosis). Complications include hypokalaemia (unable to excrete H^+; therefore preferentially excretes K^+ in the distal tubules), rickets/osteomalacia and renal stones/nephrocalcinosis.

Box 4.11 Causes of type 1 renal tubular acidosis

1. Familial (AD, AR and X-linked forms reported)
2. Associated with autoimmune disease e.g.
    Sjögren syndrome
    SLE
    AICAH
    PBC
3. Associated with nephrocalcinosis e.g.
    1° hyperparathyroidism
    Vitamin D intoxication
    Medullary sponge kidney
4. Associated with distal tubular damage e.g.
    Obstructive nephropathy
    Reflux nephropathy
    Papillary necrosis
5. Drugs e.g. amphotericin
6. Miscellaneous e.g. hypergammaglobulinaemia

4.17

a) Pyloric stenosis (as a result of ulcer and scarring at pylorus) with recurrent vomiting.

b) The K^+ will be low because of metabolic alkalosis.

c) Gastric outflow obstruction, caused by pyloric stenosis, with recurrent vomiting produces a metabolic alkalosis due to loss of H^+ in the vomitus. In adults this is usually caused by an ulcer in the pyloric canal. The paCO$_2$ is slightly elevated as a result of attempts at respiratory compensation whilst the K$^+$ will be low since it will be excreted in preference to H$^+$ in the distal tubule as the kidney attempts to conserve H$^+$.

4.18

a) Compensated hyperchloraemic (normal anion gap) metabolic acidosis caused by severe diarrhoea.

b) Renal tubular acidosis, ureterosigmoidostomy, pancreatic fistula (for a list of other causes see introductory notes at beginning of this section).

Although one would normally expect the potassium to be high or high normal rather than low in the presence of an acidosis, the diarrhoea will have caused potassium loss in this instance.

4.19

a) A normal anion gap (hyperchloraemic) metabolic acidosis with a low K$^+$ is strongly suggestive of renal tubular acidosis. In this case it is probably type 2 as a low renal threshold for glucose implies a proximal tubular defect.

b) Fanconi syndrome needs to be excluded in view of the glycosuria. The other causes of type 2 RTA are shown in Box 4.12.

c) Bicarbonate loading test to show high urinary bicarbonate excretion.

d) Measure the urinary concentration of amino acids, phosphate, bicarbonate and glucose to exclude Fanconi syndrome.

In type 2 renal tubular acidosis (proximal tubule) the principal abnormality is impaired bicarbonate reabsorption from the proximal tubule. In this type of RTA reabsorption of some bicarbonate still occurs in the distal tubule. As the plasma bicarbonate concentration falls, less bicarbonate is filtered at the kidney and, when the concentration falls to about 14 mmol/L, complete reabsorption of the filtered load can be achieved resulting in a normal urine pH. In addition, distal excretion of H$^+$ is unimpaired. This means that under conditions of severe acidosis acidification of the urine can still occur and the NH$_4$Cl acid load test is therefore normal in type 2 RTA. Diagnosis therefore requires that the bicarbonate load test (NaHCO$_3$) is given and urinary bicarbonate excretion is measured. In the normal person the urine is almost bicarbonate free since bicarbonate is almost completely reabsorbed. But in type 2 RTA > 15% of filtered load is excreted. (In type 1 RTA: ≅ 5% of filtered load is excreted). Osteomalacia, renal stones and nephrocalcinosis are rare; an equilibrium is reached where all of the filtered bicarbonate can be reabsorbed, therefore additional buffering from bone is not necessary.

Box 4.12 Causes of type 2 renal tubular acidosis

1. Familial (AD)
2. As part of Fanconi syndrome
3. Paraproteinaemia
4. Heavy metal poisoning
5. Hyperparathyroidism
6. Wilson's disease
7. Acetazolamide therapy (carbonic anhydrase inhibitor)

4.20

a) Plasma salicylate levels.

b) Accidental salicylate overdose.

Metabolic acidosis predominates in children whereas in adults a respiratory alkalosis is the initial abnormality, followed by a mixed respiratory alkalosis-metabolic acidosis, and finally a metabolic acidosis. Salicylates can give a false positive result with clinitest (but not clinistix which is specific for glucose).

4.21

a) Hyperchloraemic (normal anion gap) metabolic acidosis.

The patient's apparent shortness of breath is caused by hyperventilation as he attempts to compensate for the acidosis by 'blowing off' CO_2.

b) Acetazolamide, which is a carbonic anhydrase inhibitor used in the treatment of glaucoma, can cause renal tubular acidosis (type 2).

Type 4 renal tubular acidosis

Caused by aldosterone deficiency or resistance to action of aldosterone, therefore [K^+] is high.

Box 4.13 Causes of type 4 renal tubular acidosis	
1. Hypoaldosteronism e.g.	Addison's disease
2. Hyporeninaemia e.g.	Diabetes NSAIDs
3. Distal tubule disease e.g.	Obstructive nephropathy Papillary necrosis (e.g. sickle-cell disease)
4. K^+ sparing diuretics e.g.	Amiloride Spironolactone

5 RHEUMATOLOGY

Table 5.1 Autoantibodies associated with rheumatic diseases

Autoantibody	Associated disease	Incidence positive
Rheumatoid factor	• RA	70–80%
	• Sjögren syndrome	~100%
	• Felty syndrome	~100%
	• Mixed cryoglobulinaemia	90–100%
	• PBC	50–70%
	• MCTD	50%
	• Infective endocarditis	< 50%
	• SLE	< 40%
	• Sarcoid	30%
	• Systemic sclerosis	< 30%
	• CAH	25–40%
	• Acute viral infections	15–65%
	• Normals	5–10%
Anti-nuclear antibodies (these include anti-nucleic acid, anti-histone, anti-extractable nuclear antigen, and anti-Jo1 antibodies)	• SLE	95%
	• Juvenile RA	75%
	• AICAH	75%
	• Sjögren syndrome	70%
	• Systemic sclerosis	65%
	• Rheumatoid arthritis	30–40%
	• Polymyositis	25%
	• Normals	0–2%
Anti-nucleic acid antibodies		
Anti-dsDNA	• SLE	50%
Anti-ssDNA	• Drug-induced SLE	80%
	• SLE	70%
Anti-ENA antibodies		
Anti-sm	• SLE	30%
Anti-RNP	• MCTD	95%
	• SLE	30–40%
Anti-SSA (anti-Ro)	• Sjögren syndrome	60–70%
	• SLE	30–40%
Anti-SSB (anti-LA)	• Sjögren syndrome	40–60%
	• SLE	15%
Anti-Scl-70	• Scleroderma	70%
Anti-centromere	• CREST syndrome	80%
Anti-Jo1 antibody	• Polymyositis	30%
	• Dermatomyositis	5%
Anti-smooth muscle antibody	• AICAH	40–90%
	• PBC	30–70%
	• Idiopathic cirrhosis	25–30%
	• Viral infections (low titres)	80%
	• Normals	~10%
Anti-histone antibody	• Drug-induced SLE	95%
	• SLE	30–70%
	• RA	15–20%
Anti-neutrophil cytoplasmic antibody		
cANCA (PR3-ANCA)	• Wegener's granulomatosis	85%
pANCA (MPO-ANCA)	• Microscopic polyangiitis	80%
	• Churg–Strauss syndrome	70%
Anti-GBM antibody	• Goodpasture syndrome	90%

RA = rheumatoid arthritis; PBC = primary biliary cirrhosis; MCTD = mixed connective tissue disease; SLE = systemic lupus erythematosus; CAH = chronic active hepatitis; AICAH = autoimmune chronic active hepatitis; GBM = glomerular basement membrane

RHEUMATOLOGY

VASCULITIS

Table 5.2 Classification and causes of the systemic vasculitides

Classification	Principal vessels affected	Causes († = associated with ANCA) Granulomatous	Non-granulomatous
Large vessel	Large arteries including aorta	• Giant cell arteritis • Takayasu's arteritis	
Medium-sized vessel	Arteries (excluding aorta)		• Polyarteritis nodosa • Kawasaki's disease
Small vessel	Arterioles, capillaries and venules mainly but arteries may also be involved	• Wegener's granulomatosis† • Churg–Strauss syndrome†	• Microscopic polyangiitis† • Henoch–Schönlein purpura • Essential cryoglobulinaemia • Lupus vasculitis • Rheumatoid vasculitis • Behçet's disease • Goodpasture syndrome • Infection-induced vasculitis • Drug-induced vasculitis • Paraneoplastic vasculitis • Cutaneous leukocytoclastic vasculitis

Anti-neutrophil cytoplasmic antibody (ANCA)

These are antibodies that react with neutrophil cytoplasm; historically, they have been divided into cANCA and pANCA, based on the pattern of indirect immunofluorescence produced when patient's sera is added to immobilized neutrophils. More recently, however, immunological assays have demonstrated that the same pattern of immunofluorescence may be produced by antibodies of more than one specificity and these antibody types may now be measured directly.

cANCA gives a cytoplasmic pattern of immunofluorescence and most commonly (> 90%) has antibody specificity for proteinase 3, a serine protease. It is highly specific for Wegener's granulomatosis and 85% of patients with active Wegener's will be cANCA positive.

pANCA gives a perinuclear pattern of immunofluorescence. There are several types of pANCA, each with specificity for a different molecule, but pANCA directed against myeloperoxidase is the most common (90%). pANCA may be found in a number of different vasculitides but it is most strongly associated with microscopic polyangiitis (where it is found in 80% of cases) and Churg–Strauss syndrome (where it is found in 70%). It may also be found in a number of other conditions, particularly chronic inflammatory gastrointestinal diseases such as Crohn's disease, ulcerative colitis, primary sclerosing cholangitis and chronic active hepatitis.

5.1

See also question 7.7

a) Wegener's granulomatosis.

b) ANCA levels and renal biopsy with histological examination and immunofluorescence of the tissue specimen are the tests of choice. Histological examination of a nasal biopsy specimen is an alternative to renal biopsy but is more likely to just show non-specific necrosis rather than diagnostic changes.

Wegener's granulomatosis is a necrotizing, granulomatous vasculitis of small vessels that classically affects the upper and/or lower respiratory tract together with the kidneys (upper and lower respiratory tract granulomas with necrotizing glomerulonephritis). However it is a multi-system disease and any organ can be affected by vasculitis, resulting in a wide range of presentations dependent upon the principal sites involved. The combination of upper and/or lower respiratory tract signs or symptoms together with renal impairment should always lead one to suspect Wegener's granulomatosis (in this case red cells and red cell casts in the urine are evidence of renal vasculitis). Chronic sinusitis is a well-recognized presentation and diplopia can also occur through involvement of extraocular muscles, palsies of the III, IV or VI nerves or direct restriction of ocular movement by a retro-orbital pseudotumour (mass of granulomatous tissue).

cANCA (see p. 217) is highly specific for Wegener's granulomatosis (for the purposes of the MRCP exam) and is positive in over 85% of untreated cases. Histological evidence is also usually sought and renal biopsy is the usual method of achieving this, although transbronchial biopsy is also used and biopsy of the nasal mucosa may be useful if upper respiratory tract symptoms are present. Renal biopsy specimens should undergo both histological and immunofluorescence examination since the same histological changes (focal segmental necrosis of capillary walls) and clinical picture can be caused by other systemic small vessel vasculitides such as SLE, Henoch–Schönlein purpura (HSP), Goodpasture syndrome, mixed cryoglobulinaemia and microscopic polyangiitis. On immunofluorescence the vasculitis of SLE characteristically shows glomerular and extraglomerular deposits of IgG, IgM and complement, that of HSP shows mesangial deposits of IgA, Goodpasture syndrome shows linear deposits of IgG along the basement membrane, and mixed cryoglobulinaemia shows granular subendothelial deposits of IgG and C3. The vasculitis of Wegener's granulomatosis and microscopic polyangiitis (and Churg–Strauss syndrome) is characteristically 'pauci-immune', meaning that there is very little in the way of immunofluorescence staining. Differentiation of Wegener's from microscopic polyangiitis depends on the exact clinical picture; measurement of ANCA (Wegener's is characteristically cANCA positive whereas microscopic polyangiitis is characteristically pANCA positive, although both of these conditions are ANCA negative in about 10% of cases so a negative test for ANCA does not exclude the diagnosis); and histology of other tissue e.g. nasal or transbronchial biopsy (granulomas are not seen in microscopic polyangiitis).

Rheumatoid factor is positive in 50% of patients with Wegener's. The anaemia is likely to be normochromic and normocytic, and is caused by chronic disease. A polyclonal increase in immunoglobulins is a non-specific change that occurs in a number of inflammatory conditions, including infection, vasculitis and rheumatological conditions.

5.2

a) Mixed cryoglobulinaemia secondary to chronic HCV infection.

b) Serum cryoglobulins should be measured in order to confirm the diagnosis. A renal biopsy should also be obtained for histological examination and immunofluorescence staining in order to confirm renal involvement and assess extent of involvement since this will determine how aggressively the disease needs to be treated (it may also exclude cryoglobulinaemia as a cause of the renal impairment, in which case another cause would need to be sought). Liver biopsy with histological examination should also be performed to assess whether cirrhosis is present since this is one of the factors that determines whether α-interferon treatment for the HCV infection is appropriate.

The presence of a purpuric rash indicates that cutaneous vasculitis is present. In addition this patient has low C3 and C4 and impaired renal function, which could be indicative of glomerulonephritis (for the causes of GN associated with low complement see Box 4.3). Unexplained reduction C4 with renal/skin disease should always be investigated for cryoglobulinaemia. HCV is strongly associated with mixed cryoglobulinaemia (particularly type II) and the presence of HCV DNA, which indicates viral replication and hence active HCV infection, therefore further supports the diagnosis of mixed cryoglobulinaemia. One would also expect to see a positive rheumatoid factor since the cryoglobulins contain immunoglobulins with rheumatoid factor activity. The elevated liver enzymes may be secondary to chronic active hepatitis from HCV infection or caused by vasculitis affecting the liver.

Cryoglobulins interfere with the routine immunochemical assays used to measure serum immunoglobulins and can result in spuriously low levels as seen in this case. They may also result in spurious leukocytosis/thrombocytosis through interference with automated Coulter counters. Blood should therefore be collected and analysed at 37°C to avoid such errors.

5.3

a) Polyarteritis nodosa.

b) Henoch–Schönlein purpura.

c) Biopsy of affected skin for histological examination and immunofluorescence staining; mesenteric angiogram and serum IgA are all indicated.

The presence of purpura together with a very high ESR means that vasculitis affecting the small or medium-sized

RHEUMATOLOGY

vessels is highly probable. Absence of rheumatoid factor makes essential cryoglobulinaemia unlikely; absence of ANA makes SLE unlikely; and absence of ANCA makes Wegener's unlikely and microscopic polyangiitis or Churg–Strauss syndrome less likely. Since the clinical picture does not fit with the other causes of small or medium-sized vessel vasculitis, polyarteritis nodosa (PAN) or Henoch–Schönlein purpura (HSP) are the diagnoses that remain. The extent of the constitutional symptoms is too great and the duration of the symptoms is a little too long to be characteristic of HSP which (apart from the renal lesions) usually settles within 4–6 weeks. In addition the temporal relationship of the abdominal pain to meals is suggestive of mesenteric ischaemia (mesenteric angina), which is more typical of PAN than HSP. HBV infection is associated with 30% of cases of PAN and the presence of HbsAg therefore further supports this diagnosis.

Biopsy of skin lesions will show infiltration of the walls of small and medium-sized arteries with neutrophils in PAN whereas immunofluorescence staining will show deposits of IgA and C3 in the walls of capillaries and arterioles in HSP. Mesenteric angiography will show alternating aneurysms and stenosis in PAN (string of beads appearance). IgA is raised in 50% of cases of HSP.

5.4

a) Giant cell (cranial or temporal) arteritis.

b) Patients with giant cell arteritis (GCA) are at risk of blindness through involvement of the ciliary arteries producing optic neuritis and therefore treatment with high dose corticosteroids (for example 60 mg prednisolone) should be started immediately.

c) Diagnosis of giant cell arteritis is largely clinical, but one should always seek to confirm the diagnosis by histological examination of a temporal artery biopsy (this is the only test that is specific for giant cell arteritis). However, since the arteritis is patchy, a negative biopsy should not detract from the diagnosis if the clinical suspicion is high.

d) Anaemia of chronic disease is common in GCA.

Myalgia and malaise occur in a number of conditions (Box 5.1) but most commonly accompany infections, particularly viral infections. The duration of symptoms in this case, however, make a viral or acute bacterial aetiology unlikely and negative blood cultures make a more chronic bacterial infection such as infective endocarditis unlikely. The presence of a very high ESR means that an inflammatory or malignancy-related cause is probable but this still leaves a wide differential diagnosis, including GCA, other vasculitides, polymyalgia rheumatica, polymyositis, SLE and a number of malignancies. The presence of a persistent headache is highly suggestive of GCA and the history of jaw and tongue claudication is pathognomonic of this condition. The presence of a normal CK makes polymyositis unlikely.

Box 5.1 Causes of polymyalgia

1. Infection
    Viral
    Bacterial
2. Malignancy
    Myeloma
    Leukaemia or lymphoma
    Metastatic cancer
3. Polymyalgia rheumatica/giant cell arteritis
4. Rheumatic disease
    Osteoarthritis
    Rheumatoid arthritis
    Connective tissue disease
5. Polymyositis/dermatomyositis
6. Metabolic disease
    Hypothyroidism
    Osteomalacia
7. Other
    Fibromyalgia
    Parkinson's disease

5.5

a) Anti-neutrophil cytoplasmic antibody, anti-glomerular basement membrane antibody and renal biopsy with immunofluorescence staining of the specimen are all indicated.

RHEUMATOLOGY

b) Goodpasture syndrome.

Goodpasture syndrome is the combination of rapidly progressive glomerulonephritis, alveolar haemorrhage and anti-glomerular basement membrane (anti-GBM) antibodies, although anti-GBM antibodies are not found in 10% of cases. Glomerulonephritis associated with anti-GBM antibodies can also occur without lung disease and in this case it is classed generically as an anti-glomerular basement membrane disease rather than Goodpasture. Lung haemorrhage is strongly associated with smoking (rare in non-smokers).

This patient has pulmonary haemorrhage and renal impairment. The causes of pulmonary–renal syndrome are shown in Box 7.2, p. 258. Absence of constitutional symptoms makes a systemic vasculitis (such as Wegener's, Churg–Strauss, MPA) or Legionnaire's disease unlikely and the chest X-ray does not show any evidence of bronchial tumour; thus Legionnaire's disease remains as the most likely cause.

Although systemic vasculitis is unlikely, this diagnosis still needs to be excluded and both cANCA and pANCA should therefore be measured. Anti-GBM antibody is positive in 90% of cases of Goodpasture and immunofluorescence shows linear deposits of IgG ± C3 along the glomerular basement membrane.

5.6

a) Aortogram to demonstrate segmental vasculitis.

b) Takayasu's disease.

The presence of a widened aortic arch is suggestive of an aortic arch aneurysm, and aortic regurgitation is supportive of this diagnosis. The causes of an aortic arch aneurysm are shown in Box 5.2 but the elevated ESR suggests that aortitis is the underlying cause. A negative test for rheumatoid factor makes RA unlikely and negative VDRL and TPHA exclude syphilis. The discrepancy in BP between the right and left arms suggests that the branches of the aorta (i.e. the left subclavian artery) are also involved, which is not a feature of aortitis associated with the spondyloarthropathies. Although giant cell arteritis can cause an aortic arch syndrome, this is not usual and giant cell arteritis is rare

> **Box 5.2 Causes of aortic arch aneurysm**
> 1. Marfan syndrome
> 2. Pseudoxanthoma elasticum
> 3. Ehlers–Danlos syndrome
> 4. Aortitis
>   Syphilis
>   Spondyloarthropathies
>   RA
>   Takayasu's disease
>   Giant cell arteritis

below the age of 50. Takayasu's disease is therefore the most likely diagnosis.

Takayasu's disease (also known as 'aortic arch syndrome' and 'pulseless disease') is most commonly found in young Oriental females. It is a large vessel vasculitis, of unknown aetiology, that principally affects the aorta and its branches (particularly the proximal parts) although the pulmonary artery is also often involved. Involvement of the renal arteries commonly results in hypertension.

CONNECTIVE TISSUE DISEASES

The connective tissue (collagen vascular) diseases form a group of overlapping conditions that share certain features in common, for example autoimmune pathogenesis (probably), Raynaud's, vasculitis, multi-system involvement and positive tests for autoantibodies (Table 5.1). They include SLE (Q 4.5), systemic sclerosis (Q 5.7), dermatomyositis/polymyositis (Q 6.8), mixed connective tissue disease, the primary vasculitides (Table 5.2 and Qs 5.1–5.6), rheumatoid arthritis (Q 5.8) and relapsing polychondritis.

An overlap syndrome is said to be present if the patient has features of > 1 connective tissue disease. The commonest overlaps are systemic sclerosis/polymyositis, SLE/rheumatoid arthritis and systemic sclerosis/SLE. Mixed connective tissue disease is the term used to describe the overlap of systemic sclerosis/SLE/polymyositis and is associated with anti-U_1RNP antibodies. A few patients have insufficient features to be adequately categorized and are termed 'undifferentiated connective tissue syndrome'. Many of these develop features characteristic of one of the connective tissue disorders over

5.7

See also questions 4.5 and 6.8

a) Limited cutaneous systemic sclerosis (CREST syndrome).

b) CREST is an acronym for **C**alcinosis (subcutaneous, particularly affecting the finger pads), **R**aynaud syndrome, **E**sophageal [American spelling] dysmotility, **S**clerodactyly and **T**elangiectasia. Raynaud is already present (the classical sequence of colour changes in digits produced by exposure to cold and caused by constriction of digital arteries: pallor followed by cyanosis followed by flushing ± pain).

Box 5.3 Causes of Raynaud syndrome

Idiopathic (95%)

Secondary (5%)

1. Collagen vascular diseases
   Systemic sclerosis, SLE, polymyositis/dermatomyositis, RA, MCTD, vasculitis
2. Haematological disorders
   Cryoglobulinaemia, cold agglutinins, polycythaemia, thrombocythaemia, monoclonal gammopathies (especially Waldenström)
3. Arterial disease
   Atherosclerosis, thromboangiitis obliterans, embolic disease
4. Neurovascular compression
   Thoracic outlet syndrome, carpal tunnel syndrome
5. Use of vibrating tools
6. Malignancy
7. Drugs
   Ergotamine, β-blockers

---

c) Nail fold capillary microscopy is characteristically abnormal and shows dilated capillary loops (a mixture of giant loops and avascular areas is characteristic of diffuse cutaneous disease).

Raynaud and puffy (sausage-shaped) fingers are the classical presentation of systemic sclerosis (or one of the overlap syndromes/mixed connective tissue disease). The other features of the disease come on after a varying period of time, depending upon the subtype of systemic sclerosis that is present. Positive anti-centromere antibody is characteristic of the limited cutaneous subtype (otherwise known as CREST syndrome) whereas a positive anti-topoisomerase 1 antibody (otherwise known as anti-Scl-70) would be characteristic of the diffuse cutaneous subtype. The negative test for anti-RNP antibody makes mixed connective tissue disease or one of the overlap syndromes unlikely.

Box 5.4 The spectrum of sclerodermoid diseases

Systemic sclerosis
  Limited cutaneous
  Diffuse cutaneous
  Scleroderma sine scleroderma

Localized scleroderma (skin only involved; rarely progress to systemic involvement)
  Morphoea (dermal, subcutaneous and pansclerotic variants)
  Linear scleroderma
  Generalized morphoea

Chemicals implicated in the development of scleroderma
  Silica (stonemasons, miners; breast implants unproven and controversial)
  Alanine-treated rapeseed oil (toxic oil syndrome)
  Epoxy resins
  Organic chemicals (vinyl chloride, trichloroethylene, benzene, toluene)
  Drugs (5-hydroxytryptophan, bromocriptine, bleomycin, appetite suppressants, pentazocin, cocaine)

5.8

a) Rheumatoid arthritis.

b) Felty syndrome consists of RA, splenomegaly and neutropenia (± anaemia ± thrombocytopenia).

c) Splenomegaly.

d) Secondary Sjögren syndrome.

e) X-ray of the hands and wrists to show synovial thickening and erosions affecting the small joints (evidence of RA); Schirmer's test (to confirm keratoconjunctivitis sicca); and histological examination of a minor salivary gland biopsy (to show inflammatory infiltrate and fibrosis supporting diagnosis of Sjögren) are all indicated. Bone marrow aspirate and biopsy is also indicated in view of the neutropenia but is not a diagnostic test as such.

Patients with Sjögren syndrome often complain of a gritty sensation in the eyes or uncomfortable contact lenses because of deficient tear production. In addition, reduced saliva production results in difficulty with chewing and swallowing together with increased susceptibility to oral candidiasis. The presence of anti-SSA (anti-Ro) antibodies supports this diagnosis. Pain and stiffness affecting the small joints of the hand comprise one of the commonest presentations of RA, but can also occur in a number of other rheumatic conditions, as can a positive test for rheumatoid factor. However, most cases of secondary Sjögren syndrome occur in RA so this remains the most likely diagnosis. Felty syndrome complicates about 1% of cases of RA.

Keratoconjunctivitis sicca can be confirmed objectively by Schirmer's test (one end of a strip of filter paper is placed behind the lower eyelid and the distance along the paper that tears are absorbed is measured after 5 min – < 10 mm is a positive test) but diagnosis should be confirmed by histological examination of a biopsy of one of the minor salivary glands (usually the labial glands behind the lower lip; histology shows a lymphocytic infiltrate surrounding the vessels and ducts with sparing of the acini – these changes are not specific, however).

SPONDYLOARTHROPATHIES

Box 5.5 Clinical features common to the spondyloarthropathies	
Articular features	
1. Spondylitis	This is the term for involvement of the spine. Severe, progressive spondylitis results in: • Bony bridges (syndesmophytes) forming between the margins of adjacent vertebrae. • Ossification of the interspinous ligaments caused by chronic enthesesitis. This, together with syndesmophyte formation, gives the spine a 'tramline' appearance on the AP X-ray. • 'Squaring' of the vertebrae, caused by erosion of their corners and most marked in the lumbar region; this can be seen on the lateral X-ray. • Romanus lesions (erosion at the upper or lower border of the vertebra), best seen on the AP X-ray.
2. Sacroiliitis	Involvement of sacroiliac joints (SIJs) is usually bilateral and mainly affects the lower anterior synovial part of the joint. Early changes include justa-articular osteoporosis and capsular enthesopathy, which causes bony overgrowth over the anterior and posterior aspect of the joint. Radiographically this is manifest as erosion of the joint surfaces with marginal sclerosis. In the later stages obliteration of the joint is seen.
3. Enthesopathy	Inflammation followed by calcification of the insertions of tendons and ligaments into bone e.g. plantar fasciitis, Achilles tendinitis, chostochondritis. Calcification leads to formation of bony spurs.
4. Peripheral arthritis	This is characteristically an asymmetrical oligoarthritis with lower limb predominance (mainly large joints although dactylitis is common, particularly of the toes).
Extra-articular features	
1. Uveitis	
2. Aortic regurgitiation (because of aortitis)	
3. Upper zone pulmonary fibrosis with cavitation (*Aspergillus* colonization may occur)	
4. Secondary amyloidosis	

The spondyloarthropathies are also known as seronegative spondyloarthropathies since they are characteristically rheumatoid factor negative. (**NB**: the seronegative arthropathies do not include seronegative rheumatoid arthritis.) Together they form a group of related and overlapping inflammatory arthritides (Box 5.6) that share

RHEUMATOLOGY

certain articular and extra-articular features (Box 5.5), have a familial tendency and are strongly associated with the class 1 histocompatability antigen HLA-B27. Despite this strong association, the majority of people with HLA-B27 do not develop one of the spondyloarthropathies and tissue typing therefore does not usually aid diagnosis.

Box 5.6   Diseases that can be classified as spondyloarthropathies

1. Ankylosing spondylitis
2. Psoriatic arthritis
3. Reiter syndrome
4. Reactive arthritis
5. Enteropathic arthritis (associated with inflammatory bowel disease)
6. Undifferentiated spondyloarthropathies
7. Whipple's disease

Other causes of arthritis that are seronegative are shown in Box 5.7.

Box 5.7   Causes of a seronegative arthritis

1. Any of the spondyloarthropathies
2. Endocarditis
3. Acromegaly
4. Lyme disease
5. Behçet's disease
6. Wilson's disease
7. Sarcoidosis
8. Sickle-cell disease
9. Haemochromatosis
10. Familial Mediterranean fever
11. Leukaemia
12. Hypertrophic pulmonary osteoarthropathy

5.9

See also question 7.4

a) Incomplete Reiter syndrome.

The high white cell content of this man's synovial fluid indicates an inflammatory arthritis. When faced with an inflammatory monoarthritis one should always have septic arthritis high on the list of differential diagnoses, and in the presence of dysuria or a urethral discharge (vaginal in women) one must consider gonococcal arthritis. However, in this case microscopy and culture are negative, which makes joint infection unlikely. Microscopy has also excluded one of the crystal arthropathies (gout or pseudogout), another common cause of monoarthritis. Reiter syndrome is the triad of arthritis, urethritis (classically urethritis, but cervicitis is also included) and conjunctivitis and classically follows infection of the genitourinary (classically *Chlamydia trachomatis* and *Neisseria gonorrhoeae*) or gastrointestinal tract (classically *Shigella* spp., *E. coli*, *Salmonella* spp., *Yersinia* spp. and *Campylobacter jejuni*). All of the features are not always present, however, in which case it is referred to as incomplete Reiter syndrome. Reiter syndrome is also associated with a number of extra-articular features (Box 5.8); these may be particularly severe in those with HIV/AIDS.

Box 5.8 Extra-articular features of reactive arthritis and Reiter syndrome

1. See features detailed in Box 5.5
2. Circinate balanitis (a painless, serpiginous penile rash)
3. Keratoderma blennorrhagicum (brown, aseptic abscesses classically on soles of feet, also on palms)
4. Mouth ulcers
5. Dystrophic nails
6. Fever (if present then septic arthritis/other infection must be excluded)

CRYSTAL ARTHROPATHIES

5.10

See also question 8.11

a) Acute gout.

b) Thiazide diuretics impair renal excretion of uric acid and are commonly associated with both exacerbation and new presentation of gout. Loop diuretics may also precipitate acute gout, but less so than thiazides.

The microscopy changes are diagnostic of gouty arthritis (Table 5.3). Although the typical presentation is with an acutely swollen MTPJ of the great toe, 25% of cases will present with acute inflammation of a different joint. The serum urate may be normal in gout.

RHEUMATOLOGY

Table 5.3 Abnormalities on analysis of synovial fluid*

	Appearance	Viscosity	WBC/ml	Predominant cell type	Crystals	Culture
Normal	Clear, colourless	High	< 200	Mononuclear	None	Sterile
Osteoarthritis	Clear, straw-coloured	High	< 5000	Mononuclear	5% have pyrophosphate	Sterile
Rheumatoid arthritis	Turbid, yellow	Reduced	10000–30000	Neutrophils	None	Sterile
Gout	Turbid, yellow	Reduced	10000–30000	Neutrophils	Needle-shaped, negatively birefringent	Sterile
Pyrophosphate arthropathy	Turbid, yellow	Reduced	10000–30000	Neutrophils	Brick-shaped, positively birefringent	Sterile
Reactive arthritis	Turbid, yellow	Reduced	10000–30000	Neutrophils	None	Sterile
Septic arthritis	Turbid, yellow	Reduced	Gonococcal ~ 14000 Non-gonococcal ~ 65000 TB ~ 25000	Neutrophils Neutrophils Neutrophils	None None None	Positive Positive Positive (but takes six weeks)

*There are many tables in textbooks quoting 'exact' numbers of white cells that will be seen in various joint conditions but these differ greatly (e.g. according to Kumar and Clark one sees 30000 white cells per ml in acute gout, whereas in the *Oxford Handbook of Clinical Medicine* the number quoted is only 10000). In reality the number of cells seen in the various conditions overlaps greatly and is subject to a great deal of inter-individual variability. In practice what the physician needs to know is 'is there evidence of inflammation?' (WBC > 2000, predominantly neutrophils). If so, is this the result of infection (bacteria present on microscopy; culture positive), crystal arthropathy (crystals seen on microscopy), or reactive arthritis?

JUVENILE ARTHRITIS

5.11

a) Systemic juvenile chronic arthritis.

The 'commoner' of the childhood conditions that can cause fever, rash, lymphadenopathy and arthritis are viral infections, rheumatic fever, endocarditis, leukaemia, Henoch–Schönlein purpura and systemic juvenile chronic arthritis. The symptoms have been present for too long to be typical of a viral infection; negative throat swab and ASOT make recent streptococcal infection and therefore rheumatic fever unlikely; negative blood cultures make endocarditis unlikely (although it could still be fungal or caused by a fastidious organism); lack of anaemia, neutropenia or thrombocytopenia makes leukaemia unlikely (nearly all childhood leukaemias are acute), and there are no other features to suggest Henoch–Schönlein purpura such as abdominal pain or haematuria. Thus the most likely diagnosis is systemic juvenile chronic arthritis (formerly known as Still's disease).

Adults may also (rarely) be affected with this form of arthritis in which case it is called adult-onset Still's disease.

Box 5.9 Diagnostic criteria for systemic juvenile chronic arthritis

1. Daily fever > 39°C
2. Arthralgia/arthritis
3. Absence of rheumatoid factor
4. Absence of ANA

Plus any two of:
  a) Leucocytosis > 15×10^9/L
  b) Maculopapular rash
  c) Serositis (e.g. pleurisy, pericarditis)
  d) Hepatomegaly
  e) Splenomegaly
  f) Generalized lymphadenopathy

5.12

a) Familial Mediterranean fever (also known as periodic disease or recurrent polyserositis).

b) AA amyloid.

c) Daily colchicine as prophylaxis against further attacks.

Recurrent abdominal pain, fever and arthritis may be caused by familial Mediterranean fever (certain ethnic groups only), Henoch–Schönlein purpura and connective tissue diseases such as SLE. However, this patient does not have a typical rash or nephritis to suggest HSP (rash and haematuria can also occur in FMF and this may initially lead to difficulty in differentiating it from HSP) and the ANA is negative, which is unusual in connective tissue diseases. In addition, one of his cousins is similarly affected suggesting a familial or autosomal pattern of inheritance. Thus FMF is the most likely diagnosis. The patient has also had pleurisy associated with one of the attacks and this too is common in FMF (and connective tissue disorders).

FMF is an autosomal recessive condition characterized by recurrent bouts of fever and serositis ($\rightarrow$ abdominal pain, arthritis, pleurisy), which typically last for 1–4 days. It affects both sexes equally, but occurs almost exclusively in non-Ashkenazi Jews, Armenians, Arabs and Turks. It is therefore mainly seen in populations surrounding the Mediterranean basin (or their descendants). Onset usually occurs before the age of 20 (50% < 10 years; 80% < 20 years; 99% < 40 years).

6 NEUROLOGY

NEUROLOGY

LUMBAR PUNCTURE
Interpretation of CSF from lumbar puncture

Table 6.1 Characteristics of normal CSF and changes in various types of meningitis

	Normal	Bacterial meningitis	Viral ('aseptic') meningitis	Tuberculous
Opening pressure	< 20 cm of CSF	↑	↑/→	↑
Appearance	Clear, colourless	Turbid	Clear/slightly turbid	Clear/ slightly turbid, ?fibrin web
Glucose	> 2/3 plasma glucose	↓	→	↓
Protein	< 0.4 g/L	↑↑	↑/→	↑
White blood cells	< 5	↑↑	↑	↑
Predominant cell type	Lymphocytes only	Neutrophils	Lymphocytes	Lymphocytes

6.1

See also questions 7.6 and 7.9

a) Bacterial meningitis.

b) Take blood for culture and give high-dose intravenous benzylpenicillin or cefotaxime.

The CSF shows an elevated white cell count consisting mainly of neutrophils. This pattern is diagnostic of bacterial meningitis until proven otherwise. The CSF glucose is low relative to the blood glucose and this is also supportive of bacterial infection. In addition, this patient's symptoms are of rapid onset (< 48 h), which is characteristic. Increased CSF protein is a non-specific sign of intracranial pathology.

Most cases of community-acquired bacterial meningitis in adults will be caused by *Neisseria meningitidis* or *Streptococcus pneumoniae* (Gram negative bacilli, *Haemophilus influenzae* and *Staphylococcus aureus* account for the majority of the remainder of cases) and the antibiotic chosen should therefore cover these organisms and penetrate the CSF well. The antibiotic of choice used to be benzylpenicillin but many hospitals now recommend cefotaxime because of increasing pneumococcal resistance to penicillin.

Remember that the classical signs of meningitis do not always occur and rash is only characteristic of meningococcal meningitis associated with septicaemia – it will not be seen in the other forms of meningitis or in meningococcal meningitis with no associated septicaemia. A high index of suspicion is therefore essential.

6.2

a) Herpes simplex encephalitis or cerebral abscess affecting the left temporal lobe.

b) CT/MRI brain with focus on temporal lobe, an EEG to look for abnormalities with a temporal lobe focus, and herpes simplex PCR of the CSF are all indicated. Electron microscopy of the CSF to look for herpes virus particles is an alternative to PCR if this test is not available.

This patient has an elevated CSF white cell count, which consists mainly of lymphocytes and the CSF glucose is low. The causes of this pattern of abnormality are shown in Box 6.1. Smelling coffee could represent olfactory hallucinations and an upper temporal quadrantic hemianopia is consistent with temporal lobe pathology. Herpes simplex has a predilection for the temporal lobes but the CSF may actually be normal in this condition. One should therefore always have a high index of suspicion in someone who presents with temporal lobe features. Treatment is with intravenous acyclovir for 10 days. One also needs to exclude a space

---

Box 6.1   Causes of aseptic* meningitis with low CSF glucose

1. Tuberculosis
2. Cerebral/spinal/extradural abscess
3. Partially treated bacterial meningitis
4. Difficult to detect bacteria e.g. spirochaetes (syphilis, Lyme disease, leptospirosis), *Brucella, Rickettsia*
5. Fungi e.g. *Cryptococcus,* histoplasmosis
6. Protozoa e.g. cerebral malaria, toxoplasmosis, amoebiasis
7. Helminths e.g. hydatid, cysticercosis
8. Malignancy e.g. meningeal metastases, acute leukaemia, cerebral lymphoma
9. Neurosarcoidosis
10. Behçet's disease
11. CNS vasculitis e.g. SLE
12. Whipple's disease

*Aseptic meningitis = CSF lymphocyte pleocytosis with no growth on standard culture media and no organisms seen on Gram stain

occupying lesion, and in view of the inflammatory CSF changes a cerebral abscess or extradural abscess lying adjacent to the temporal lobe is the most likely potential cause. The onset and progression of symptoms are too rapid for cerebral metastases or lymphoma.

6.3

a) Tuberculous meningitis.

b) SIADH.

This patient has disease of subacute onset accompanied by lesions of the VI and VII cranial nerves. Her CSF picture is characteristic of tuberculous meningitis and this condition classically presents in a subacute fashion with a few weeks of non-specific or constitutional symptoms prior to the onset of signs of meningitis. Cranial nerve lesions occur in 25% of those with tuberculous meningitis and are indicative of involvement of the basal meninges. Treatment is with rifampicin, pyrazinamide and isoniazid. HIV should be suspected in anyone presenting with TB these days.

SIADH may occur in tuberculous meningitis (and in other basal meningitides) and this complication should be suspected in view of the low sodium. Hydrocephalus caused by obstruction of the flow or reabsorption of CSF is a particular problem of tuberculous meningitis. Other complications include cerebral infarction as a result of arteritis and radiculopathy (often multiple) or myelopathy caused by spinal arachnoiditis. Any of the diseases in Box 6.1 may cause the same CSF picture as tuberculous meningitis; diagnosis therefore relies on other clinical indications of TB (CXR, positive tuberculin test, clinical picture, and so on) and upon positive cultures. In addition PCR for mycobacterium tuberculosis can now be performed on the CSF. Indian ink staining is useful for excluding cryptococcal meningitis.

6.4

a) Sporadic Creutzfeldt–Jakob disease.

Creutzfeldt–Jakob disease (CJD) is a prion disease that causes a spongiform encephalopathy. It may be sporadic, iatrogenic (for example caused by treatment with infected material such as corneal grafts or growth hormone derived from pituitary extracts) or familial (about 15% of cases have an autosomal dominant form of transmission).

Sporadic CJD is mainly found in patients between 50 and 70 years of age and presents with behavioural change, signs of dementia or focal neurological features, which may resemble those of stroke. Myoclonus is universal at some stage of the disease. The clinical course is that of rapidly progressive dementia and the mean duration of illness is about five months. There are no antemortem diagnostic tests at present other than brain biopsy, although the clinical picture of dementia, myoclonus and periodic, biphasic or triphasic synchronous sharp-wave complexes on EEG is highly suggestive. Lumbar puncture is usually normal but should be performed to exclude treatable causes of dementia such as neurosyphilis. There is no effective treatment.

Recently 'new variant Creutzfeldt–Jakob disease' has emerged and is believed to be caused by consumption of infected beef products. It occurs in a younger cohort of patients than sporadic CJD, presents with mainly neuropsychiatric disturbance and cerebellar ataxia and is not characteristically associated with myoclonus. The EEG features mentioned above are not found in this condition.

6.5

a) Partially treated bacterial meningitis.
b) Cerebral abscess.

The CSF shows an aseptic lymphocyte pleocytosis with reduced glucose. The differential diagnosis for this picture is shown in Box 6.1. However, the recent history of antibiotic treatment for URTI means that partially treated bacterial meningitis is a likely diagnosis and one should suspect pneumococcus as the infecting organism. Blood should be taken for culture in the presence of inhibitors of amoxycillin in an effort to culture the organism. Sending CSF to test for pneumococcus-specific antigen may also be helpful.

Middle ear infection is the commonest predisposing cause for cerebral abscess and this patient will therefore require a CT scan to exclude the presence of an abscess. Culture is likely to show a mixed growth of upper respiratory tract anaerobes if this is the case. Other predisposing factors to cerebral abscess include sinusitis, bacterial endocarditis, congenital heart disease with a right-to-left shunt, lung abscess/bronchiectasis and dental sepsis. In about 10% of cases no other source of infection can be found.

6.6

a) Spinal block at the level of the thoracic spine as a result of a spinal cord tumour or extradural compressive lesion (for example neurofibroma).

b) MRI scan of the brain and spinal cord is the least invasive investigation and is capable of demonstrating both the level of the tumour and its anatomical relations. It is therefore the preferred answer. CT scanning is an alternative to MRI but does not provide the same degree of detail. A myelogram could also be performed but this is invasive and will not show much in the way of anatomical detail.

c) Communicating hydrocephalus.

This patient has a very high CSF protein, the causes of which are shown in Box 6.2. Her clinical signs are of bilateral upper motor neurone lesions affecting the legs but not the arms. There is no evidence of meningitis or diabetes, the CSF red cell content is too low for subarachnoid haemorrhage and Guillain–Barré syndrome produces lower motor neurone signs only. Thus the most likely diagnosis is spinal block caused by a tumour. Normal examination of the upper limbs means that the tumour is most likely to lie below the cervical spine. The lumbar spine does not contain any upper motor neurones below the level of L1 (cauda equina only) so the thoracic spine is the most likely location.

At very high CSF protein concentrations blockage of CSF absorption at the arachnoid villi may occur causing communicating hydrocephalus. This accounts for the patient's headache and dilated ventricles. The left-sided VI nerve lesion is a false localizing sign of raised intracranial pressure.

Box 6.2 Causes of a greatly elevated CSF protein

Up to 3g/L
  Diabetic radiculopathy
  Guillain–Barré syndrome
  Myxoedema

>5g/L
  Meningitis
  Subarachnoid haemorrhage (or bloody tap)
  Spinal cord tumour with spinal block (Froin syndrome)

NEUROPHYSIOLOGY

6.7

a) Myasthenia gravis.

b) Pernicious anaemia.

c) Anti-acetylcholine receptor antibodies or a tensilon test will confirm the diagnosis.

d) CT thorax (to exclude the presence of a thymoma) and serum B12 and folate levels are indicated.

Myasthenia gravis (MG) is an organ-specific autoimmune disease associated with other organ-specific autoimmune diseases, including pernicious anaemia. It is caused by autoantibodies directed against the acetylcholine receptor of the neuromuscular junction. These autoantibodies result in progressive loss of acetylcholine receptors, which produces the clinical hallmark of muscle weakness that worsens with exercise. The eye muscles are nearly always involved (diplopia, ptosis) and involvement of skeletal muscles produces weakness and easy fatiguability, particularly affecting the proximal muscles. Involvement of the bulbar muscles results in difficulty with chewing/swallowing that gets progressively worse throughout the meal, nasal regurgitation and a snarling smile. The respiratory muscles may also be involved. An EMG showing a progressive decrement in the muscle action potential with repetitive stimulation is highly suggestive of the condition.* The presence of anti-AChR antibodies is diagnostic. A tensilon test can also be used to confirm the diagnosis in which case administration of the anti-cholinesterase edrophonium (which has a short half-life) produces a marked improvement of the symptoms that wears off after about 5 min.

In 10% of cases MG is associated with thymoma and this always needs to be excluded. It may also occur in association with penicillamine therapy but in this case the disease remits on withdrawal of the drug. Early-onset disease (< 40 years old) may improve following thymectomy. This is not the case with thymoma-associated myasthenia.

*The EMG appearance in MG contrasts with that of Eaton–Lambert myasthenic syndrome in which the amplitude of the evoked muscle potential is initially reduced but increases considerably with repetitive stimulation or following a maximum voluntary contraction. This condition is usually associated with small cell carcinoma of the lung and is caused by autoantibodies directed against pre-synaptic calcium channels.

6.8

a) Dermatomyositis.

b) Muscle biopsy and creatinine kinase.

This patient's symptoms of proximal muscle weakness are compatible with either myopathic or neurological pathology. The EMG, however, shows changes that are characteristic of myopathy (neuropathy is characterized by changes resulting from denervation: fibrillation potentials of about 1 msec duration and 50–200 µV in amplitude). The distribution of the rash is suggestive of photosensitivity and the presence of such a rash in the presence of muscle weakness should always alert the physician to the possibility of dermatomyositis. The elevated ESR is certainly compatible with an inflammatory myositis and positive tests for rheumatoid factor and ANA, although non-specific, are suggestive of a connective tissue disorder. The papules over the extensor surface of the knuckles and fingers are Gottron's papules, which are pathognomonic of dermatomyositis (a heliotrope rash over the upper eyelids is the other pathognomonic feature that may be present in dermatomyositis). The diagnosis of a polymyositis is confirmed by the following three investigations of which two should be positive:

- Elevated muscle enzymes (creatinine kinase usually measured but aldolase, LDH and serum transaminases are also elevated).
- Muscle biopsy shows muscle fibre necrosis, regeneration and atrophy with a perivascular and interstitial inflammatory infiltrate that consists mainly of lymphocytes and plasma cells.
- EMG.

The importance of dermatomyositis from an MRCP point of view lies in the fact that, in adults, it is associated with internal malignancy in about 10% (some say less) of cases. This is not the case with isolated polymyositis.

Box 6.3 Causes of proximal muscle weakness

1. Neurological
   e.g. motor neurone disease, Guillain–Barré syndrome,* nerve root compression
2. Muscular dystrophies
   e.g. limb girdle dystrophy, facioscapulohumeral dystrophy, Becker's muscular dystrophy
3. Dystrophia myotonica
4. Myasthenia gravis
5. Proximal myopathy
   e.g. Cushing syndrome, thyrotoxicosis, osteomalacia, diabetic amyotrophy (thighs only), alcoholic neuropathy (thighs only)
6. Polymyositis/dermatomyositis†
7. Eaton–Lambert syndrome†

*Guillain–Barré syndrome classically presents with distal weakness that ascends
†May be associated with malignancy

6.9

a) The features of the VEP are shown schematically in Fig. 6.8. The stimulus (usually pattern reversal on a checkerboard) is given at t = 0 and the potentials are recorded over the occipital cortex. Latency is the time taken to the first major positive deflection, the p100. The N75 and N145 are the smaller negative deflections either side of the p100 and are unimportant for MRCP purposes. The normal latency is < 110 msec. In this patient the latency in the left eye is normal but that of the right eye is delayed to 153 msec. The amplitudes are normal. These features are characteristic of demyelination of the optic nerve. Compression of the optic nerve (for example by pituitary tumour or craniopharyngioma) can also slow conduction but considerably less so than demyelination, and in the case of compression one would expect the amplitude of the VEP to be reduced.

b) Lateral rectus weakness could be caused by a primary muscle problem, or pathology affecting the VI nerve, its nucleus or central connections. Nystagmus and ataxia could be caused by a vestibular or a cerebellar lesion. All of these features could be explained by a brainstem compressive lesion such as a tumour, or brainstem vascular lesion such as a stroke, but these would not account for the optic nerve demyelination.

Multiple sclerosis (MS) is characterized by plaques of demyelination distributed throughout the CNS. It commonly affects the brainstem (internuclear ophthalmoplegia, weakness of extraocular muscles, vestibular dysfunction), cerebellum, optic nerves and spinal cord (spastic weakness and sensory loss). This is the correct unifying diagnosis.

c) Diagnosis of MS relies on demonstrating plaques of demyelination that are disseminated in time and place (that is, different areas of the CNS involved at different times).

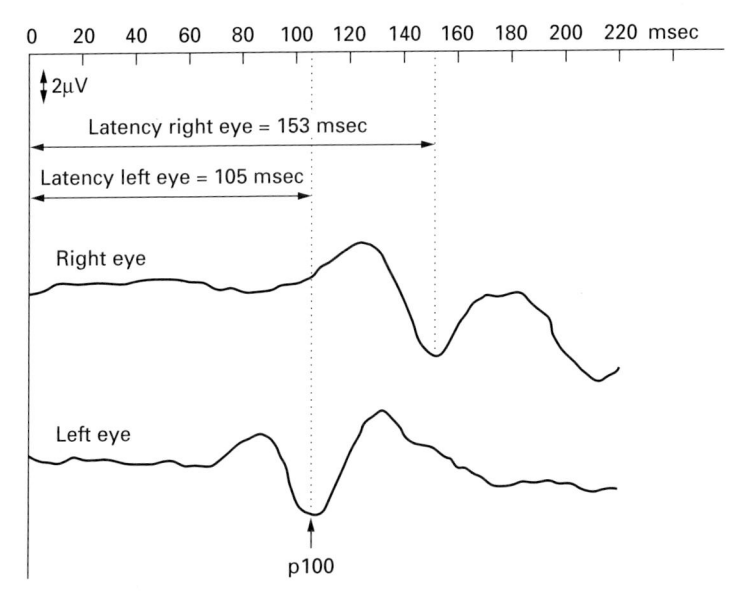

Fig. 6.8 Calculation of latency from VEP trace

Decreased latency of the VEP is evidence of previous asymptomatic optic neuritis thereby fulfilling the criterion of 'disseminated in time'. MRI of the brain and spinal cord should be performed to confirm that the current symptoms are the result of demylination (thereby fulfilling the criterion of 'disseminated in space') and to exclude the brainstem pathologies mentioned above. Examination of the CSF for oligoclonal bands (present in 90% of MS) is supportive of the diagnosis but these are non-specific.

6.10

a) 37 msec.

b) 60 msec.

c) Carpal tunnel syndrome.

Conduction velocity is calculated by dividing the distance travelled by the time taken to travel that distance. For elbow to wrist conduction this is calculated as follows:

Latency from elbow to wrist = (latency following stimulus 1)
− (latency following stimulus 2)
= 7.7 − 2.7 = 5.0 ms or 0.005 s
Distance from elbow to wrist = 30 cm or 0.3 m
Conduction velocity = 0.3/0.005 = 60 ms

Conduction velocity before the wrist is normal but after the wrist is reduced. This pattern is caused by carpal tunnel syndrome, an entrapment neuropathy produced by pressure on the median nerve as it passes under the flexor retinaculum at the wrist.

6.11

a) An axonal sensory peripheral neuropathy.

b) Causes of a predominantly sensory axonal peripheral neuropathy include diabetes mellitus (commonest cause), vitamin B_{12} deficiency, carcinoma (paraneoplastic), Sjögren syndrome and AIDS.

Peripheral neuropathies can result from axonal degeneration, demyelination or a combination of the two. In broad terms, however, axonal neuropathies are generally

NEUROLOGY

caused by metabolic, toxic or heritable causes whereas demyelinating neuropathies are generally autoimmune (inflammatory), associated with a paraproteinaemia or the result of an inherited disorder of myelin. It is very difficult to distinguish between the different types of neuropathy on clinical grounds since the same neurological deficit can be caused by either or both of the pathophysiological processes. Hence nerve conduction studies are usually required to make the distinction. Axonal neuropathies are characterized electrophysiologically by reduced amplitude of the evoked potential with a normal or only slightly reduced conduction velocity whereas in demyelinating neuropathies the opposite is true.

AUDIOLOGY

A normal audiogram is shown below. Bone conduction and air conduction should be equal (and the same in each ear) and the lines should lie at sound levels below the 20 dB mark. Zero dB is a population average so some normal patients will have traces that lie partially or completely within the negative dB portion of the graph.

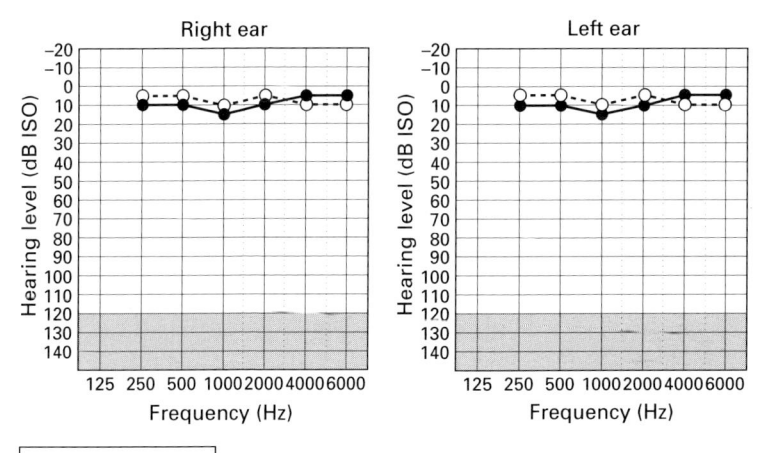

○ Air conduction
● Bone conduction

Fig. 6.9 Normal audiogram

245

6.12

a) Sensorineural deafness affecting the right ear.

b) Menière's disease.

   This patient has a normal trace in the left ear but there is impaired hearing in the right ear. This impairment affects air and bone conduction equally indicating that it is sensorineural in nature. Most causes of sensorineural deafness produce hearing loss that is more marked at higher frequencies, but the opposite is true in this patient.

   Menière's disease is a disorder that is characterized by recurrent episodes of vertigo accompanied by loud tinnitus and fluctuating sensorineural hearing loss. As time progresses the episodes of vertigo become less frequent and less severe but the deafness and tinnitus become progressively worse. It is usually unilateral but may become bilateral. There is dilation of the endolymphatic system within the membranous labyrinth and Menière's is therefore probably caused by abnormal regulation of the production, circulation and/or reabsorption of endolymph. The audiogram usually (but not always) shows sensorineural deafness that is slightly more marked at the lower frequencies.

6.13

a) Repeated acoustic trauma caused by rifle-firing.

   There is a dip at 4000 Hz on the audiogram from this patient's left ear. Bone and air conduction are equally affected indicating that it is sensorineural in nature. These dips are characteristic of noise-induced hearing loss or acoustic trauma (hearing loss through exposure to a single episode of very high intensity sound). Virtually all noise-induced hearing loss is bilateral; when firing a rifle, however, one of the ears is protected by the rifle butt and in the case of a right-handed individual this will be the right ear (the converse is true for left-handers). With continued exposure to high noise levels the 4000 Hz dips become gradually wider and the final picture is that of a sloping audiogram with progressively increasing hearing loss from low to medium to high frequencies. Subjective hearing loss is not usually reported until there is loss of > 25 dB at frequencies below 3000 Hz (at this point speech intelligibility suffers).

NEUROLOGY

6.14

a) Bilateral conductive deafness.

b) Ear wax.

The audiogram shows reduced air conduction with normal bone conduction. This pattern is characteristic of conductive deafness. The lower frequencies are affected more than the higher ones and this is also characteristic. In this patient the changes are bilateral. In a patient of this age the most likely cause of bilateral conductive deafness of relatively rapid onset is ear wax. Perforation of the tympanic membranes also causes conductive deafness but the onset of hearing loss is sudden and there should be a history of a precipitating event such as barotrauma (diving) or infection. Tumours that infiltrate the middle ear, for example nasopharyngeal carcinoma, can also cause conductive deafness of fairly rapid onset, but this would be unilateral. The conductive deafness produced by otosclerosis is insidious over several years. In a child glue ear needs to be excluded as a cause of unilateral or bilateral conductive deafness and foreign bodies are a common cause of unilateral conductive deafness.

6.15

a) CT/MRI scan of the brainstem.

b) Left-sided acoustic neuroma or meningioma compressing the cerebellar-pontine angle.

Absence of the left corneal reflex is indicative of pathology affecting the left V cranial nerve. Nystagmus to the right can be caused by a right-sided cerebellar lesion but in the presence of other left-sided pathology is more likely to result from a left-sided vestibular lesion. The audiogram shows left-sided sensorineural deafness. Thus there is pathology affecting both the auditory and the vestibular components of the VIII nerve together with the V nerve. The most likely anatomical site for this to occur is the cerebellar-pontine angle and the commonest tumour at this site is an acoustic neuroma. A non-compressive lesion is unlikely.

6.16

a) Otosclerosis.

The audiogram shows bilateral conductive deafness (bone conduction better than air conduction). However, at 2000 Hz there is a dip in the bone conduction. These are Cahart's notches and they are characteristic of otosclerosis. They do not always occur though and the audiogram may just show conductive deafness that is indistinguishable from any other cause.

Otosclerosis is a disease of unknown aetiology in which the bone of the otic capsule becomes replaced by spongy, highly vascular bone, which may then sclerose. Encroachment of this bone onto the oval window causes fixing of the stapes footplate. Onset is between the ages of 15 and 40 and females are affected twice as often as males. There is a family history in 40–50% of cases. The history is of gradually progressive conductive deafness, but tinnitus and vertigo may also occur.

7 RESPIRATORY MEDICINE

LUNG FUNCTION TESTS

Spirometry

The components of a normal spirometry trace are shown in Fig. 7.8 and the abnormalities that occur in various respiratory conditions are shown in Table 7.1.

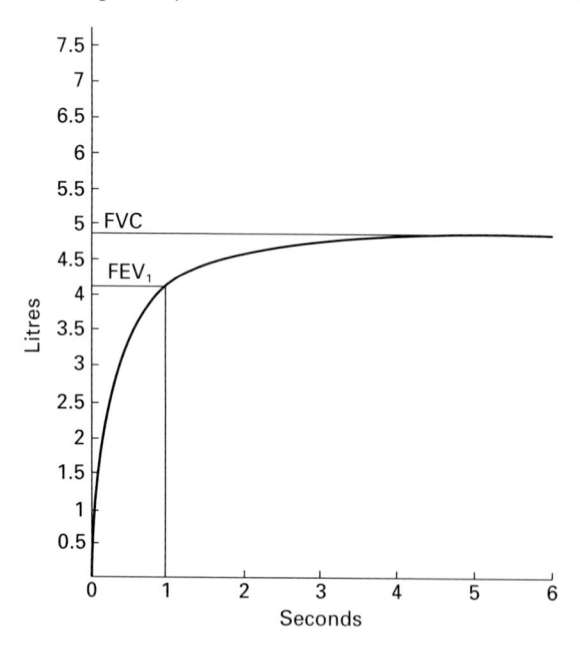

Fig. 7.8 Normal spirometry trace

Table 7.1 Abnormalities on lung function testing

	FEV_1	FVC	FEV_1/FVC	TLC	RV	T_LCO	KCO
Normal	–	–	70–80%	–	–	–	–
Interstitial lung disease (restrictive defect)	↓	↓	N/↑	↓	↓	↓	↓
Asthma (obstructive defect)	↓	↓	↓	↑	↑	N/↑	N/↑
Emphysema (obstructive defect)	↓	↓	↓	↑	↑	↓	↓

FEV_1 = forced expired volume in 1 s; FVC = forced vital capacity; TLC = total lung capacity; RV = residual volume; T_LCO = gas transfer factor for carbon monoxide (a measure of the diffusion capacity of the alveolar membranes); V_A = alveolar volume; KCO = transfer coefficient for carbon monoxide (it measures the gas transfer per unit volume of alveoli, i.e. KCO=T_LCO/V_A)

RESPIRATORY MEDICINE

Lung volumes

The components of the lung volume are shown schematically in Fig. 7.9. Tidal volume, vital capacity (VC) and inspiratory capacity (IC) can be determined from spirometry. However, residual volume (RV), and hence total lung capacity (TLC) and functional residual capacity (FRC), cannot be measured directly since the 'air' occupying this space is not exchanged during the course of a single breath. In order to measure the residual volume a helium dilution technique is used. In this technique the subject breathes in and out from a reservoir containing a known concentration of helium (a non-absorbable gas), allowing the helium to equilibrate between the container and the subject's entire lung volume. Since the concentration of helium in the reservoir is known at the start, the TLC can be calculated from the degree of dilution of the helium that has occurred. RV and FRC are then calculated as follows:

$$RV = TLC - VC$$
$$FRC = TLC - IC$$

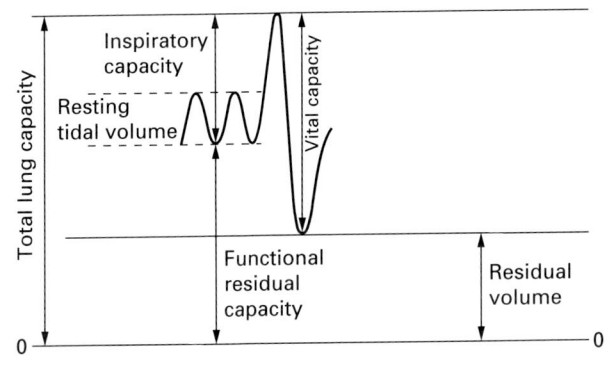

Fig. 7.9 Components of lung volume

Flow volume loops

The flow volume curve gives a measure of the volume and rate at which air flows into and out of the lungs during a forced expiration and forced inspiration (Fig. 7.10). The initial steep rise in the curve represents flow of air out of the larger airways. This is followed by a decline in the flow rate, representing air being 'squeezed' out of the smaller airways. This latter part of the curve is less effort dependent and therefore more accurately reflects the condition of the airways.

When as much air as possible has been expelled from the lungs the flow rate is nil. The volume at this point represents the FVC. The maximum point on the vertical (flow) axis represents the peak expiratory flow rate (PEFR).

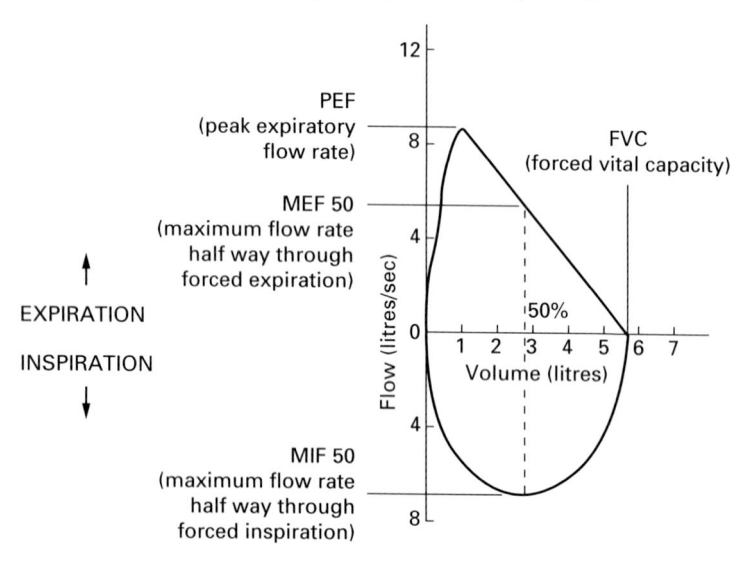

Fig. 7.10 Normal flow volume loop

Transfer factor (T_LCO or D_LCO) and transfer coefficient (KCO)

Transfer factor is a measure of the ability of a gas (carbon monoxide is used for the sake of the test) to transfer across the alveolar-capillary membrane and therefore reflects the diffusion capacity (integrity) of this membrane. The test involves inhalation of a known (but low) concentration of carbon monoxide and measurement of the amount of carbon monoxide that is 'taken up'. Transfer factor is a fairly crude measure of lung function since it is affected by blood flow (that is, V/Q relationships), haemoglobin concentration and the thickness and total surface area of alveolar membrane in the lungs. Therefore, in order to control for differences in lung volume, the T_LCO is often divided by the lung volume to give a measure of the gas transfer per unit volume of lung. This is the transfer coefficient (KCO).

Since transfer factor and transfer coefficient are dependent upon thickness of the alveolar membrane they are particularly useful for detection of, and monitoring progression of, parenchymal lung diseases such as pulmonary fibrosis.

7.1

See also questions 4.14, 4.15, 4.21 and 5.5

a) 4.0.

b) 4.8.

c) Gastro-oesophageal reflux or post-nasal drip.

d) Serial monitoring of peak expiratory flow rate.

The commonest causes of nocturnal cough are asthma, gastro-oesophageal reflux (irritation of the lower oesophagus, produces a vagal-induced reflex cough) and post-nasal drip. In this case the FEV_1, FVC and FEV_1/FVC are all normal (that is, this is a normal spirometry trace) and although this does not exclude a diagnosis of mild asthma (since the changes may be intermittent) it does suggest that an alternative diagnosis may be the cause of the nocturnal symptoms.

Because asthma is a reversible condition, one must remember that normal lung function tests are still compatible with a diagnosis of asthma. Asthma therefore still needs to be excluded and most physicians would seek to do this prior to proceeding to more invasive tests such as oesophageal pH monitoring. Pre- and post-bronchodilator lung function or serial monitoring of the peak flow rate over a few weeks should be sufficient to demonstrate the variability in airflow limitation that is characteristic of asthma. Asthma is confirmed by variations in the PEFR by more than 25% (or a 25% increase in the PEFR or FEV_1 following administration of a bronchodilator). If this is equivocal then a methacholine bronchial challenge test may be necessary to demonstrate bronchial hyperresponsiveness and thereby confirm or refute the diagnosis of asthma. However, the alternative diagnoses may be pursued prior to subjecting the patient to this potentially dangerous test.

7.2

a) Moderate/severe asthma or chronic obstructive pulmonary disease (with little emphysematous component).

b) Repeat the test after administration of an inhaled bronchodilator.

The PEFR is reduced and the downward slope of the expiratory curve is concave in appearance (that is, the MEF_{50} is reduced) indicating that airways obstruction is present. The differential diagnosis is therefore either asthma or chronic obstructive pulmonary disease. However, a more marked deformation of the downward portion of the curve would be expected if there was a significant emphysematous component to the airways disease (see Q 7.12).

An increase in the PEFR by more than 25% and improvement in the shape of the curve following administration of a β_2-agonist would indicate that the obstructive airways disease is reversible and therefore favour a diagnosis of asthma. But in reality many cases of COPD have a reversible element to them and may therefore show a degree of improvement as well.

7.3

a) Polycythaemia.

The only abnormality of lung function is increased gas transfer (T_LCO and KCO) and polycythaemia is the only haematological condition that produces this abnormality.

b) Primary proliferative polycythaemia (polycythaemia rubra vera [PCRV] in old nomenclature).

The causes of polycythaemia are shown in Box 3.2. Chronic lung disease and PCRV are the two commonest causes but, since normal spirometry makes significant lung disease unlikely, PCRV is left as the likely diagnosis (see also answer to Q 3.2).

c) Pulmonary embolus (thrombotic events, caused by the presence of polycythaemia or thrombocythaemia, may complicate the myeloproliferative disorders).

d) Polycythaemia, asthma, intra-alveolar haemorrhage (e.g. Goodpasture syndrome; Wegener's granulomatosis; pulmonary haemosiderosis) and left to right shunting of blood can all cause increased gas transfer (T_LCO and KCO).

7.4

a) Restrictive ventilatory defect.
b) Pulmonary fibrosis, kyphosis and restriction of chest wall movement as a result of ankylosis of the costovertebral and costotransverse joints.
c) Ankylosing spondylitis.

The flow volume loop shows reduced FEV_1 and FVC with a normal FEV_1/FVC ratio and an almost normal shape. This pattern is characteristic of a restrictive ventilatory defect. One would also expect to see reduced compliance. Ankylosing spondylitis is characterized by sacroiliitis (hence the low back pain) and progressive kyphosis together with ankylosis of the costovertebral and costotransverse joints. The kyphosis and ankylosis result in mechanical restriction of chest wall movement and therefore produce a restrictive ventilatory defect. Ankylosing spondylitis may also be associated with upper zone pulmonary fibrosis and cavitation (in about 1% of cases) and when present this further contributes to ventilatory restriction. If fibrosis is present the KCO will also be reduced through impaired gas exchange at the level of the alveolar membrane.

> **Box 7.1 Causes of a restrictive ventilatory defect**
>
> 1. **Restriction within the lungs caused by:**
>   a) Pulmonary fibrosis e.g.
>   Fibrosing alveolitis
>   Asbestosis
>   Autoimmune disease
>   Ankylosing spondylitis
>   Renal tubular acidosis
>   b) Pulmonary infiltration e.g.
>   Sarcoidosis
>   Lymphangitis carcinomatosis
> 2. **Restriction within the pleura e.g.**
>   Pleural thickening
>   Mesothelioma
> 3. **Restriction of chest wall caused by:**
>   a) Skeletal deformity e.g. scoliosis
>   b) Ankylosis e.g. ankylosing spondylitis
>   c) Neuromuscular weakness e.g.
>   Motor neurone disease
>   Guillain–Barré syndrome
>   Polio

7.5

a) An obstructive ventilatory defect is indicated by the combination of low FEV_1, low FVC and low FEV_1/FVC ratio. There is also air trapping (indicated by the high residual volume and total lung capacity) and reduced alveolar volume.

b) The combination of an obstructive defect with air trapping is characteristic of emphysema. One would also expect to see reduced T_LCO and KCO due to alveolar destruction.

7.6

a) Guillain–Barré syndrome.

b) Nerve conduction studies and an MRI scan of the cervical and thoracic spine are indicated.

c) Mechanical ventilation should be initiated if the FVC falls below 1.5 litres. Hypoxia ($PO_2 < 10\,kPa$) or increasing hypercapnoea ($PCO_2 > 6\,kPa$) are also criteria for ventilation.

The vitalograph shows reduced FVC with an elevated FEV_1/FVC ratio, that is, a restrictive ventilatory defect, the causes of which include neuromuscular weakness (Box 7.1).

RESPIRATORY MEDICINE

This patient's symptoms are compatible with a motor neuropathy and given the time course of progression and the temporal relationship to an enteric infection (*Campylobacter jejuni* is a recognized cause of Guillain–Barré syndrome) Guillain–Barré syndrome (GBS) is the likely diagnosis.

GBS is classically described as being a post-infectious demyelinating polyneuropathy (polyradiculopathy) although it may occur after surgery and 40% of cases are idiopathic. Infection normally precedes the development of neuropathy by about 1–3 weeks.

Symptoms develop rapidly over a period ranging from a few days to a maximum of four weeks and conform to an ascending, predominantly motor neuropathy with weakness and loss/reduction of tendon reflexes. Proximal muscles are characteristically affected to a greater degree than distal ones (in contrast to other forms of neuropathy). Cranial nerve palsies (especially VII) may occur and can result in bulbar paralysis or even 'locked in' syndrome. Respiratory muscle weakness may necessitate mechanical ventilation. Sensory symptoms include peripheral paraesthesia and lumbar or interscapular pain and may precede the motor weakness. Sensory loss may occur but is often difficult to detect. Autonomic dysfunction may also occur and can produce bladder atony, paralytic ileus, hypertension (possibly caused by denervation of the carotid sinus) and orthostatic hypotension.

Diagnosis is confirmed by nerve conduction studies which show the characteristic changes of demyelination (see Q 6.11).

7.7

a) The patient has evidence of intra-alveolar haemorrhage (haemoptysis and ill-defined shadows on CXR together with a raised T_LCO), nephritis (haematuria), and a vasculitic rash. Churg–Strauss syndrome is the most likely diagnosis in view of the eosinophilia and past history of asthma.

b) Wegener's granulomatosis or polyarteritis nodosa can also cause this clinical picture. Goodpasture syndrome can cause pulmonary haemorrhage and nephritis but is not associated with a vasculitic rash.

c) ANCA, urine microscopy and culture, skin biopsy, renal biopsy and creatinine clearance are all indicated.

Churg–Strauss syndrome is classically described as the triad of late-onset asthma, peripheral blood eosinophilia (> 10% eosinophils in the blood) and systemic vasculitis, although upper airways disease such as allergic rhinitis and sinusitis are now recognized as a part of the clinical syndrome. It is thought to be a variant of polyarteritis nodosa. The kidneys are involved but far less frequently than with other small vessel vasculitides. Involvement of the heart accounts for over 50% of deaths.

Three stages of the disease have been described: 1) allergic rhinitis ± sinusitis and asthma that becomes progressively more difficult to treat; 2) peripheral blood eosinophilia with eosinophilic pulmonary infiltrates and worsening asthma; and 3) systemic vasculitis. The diagnosis is usually made in the fourth decade and males are affected slightly more frequently than females. Churg–Strauss syndrome is extremely responsive to corticosteroids and these form the mainstay of treatment.

Box 7.2 Causes of pulmonary–renal syndromes (i.e. haemoptysis plus haematuria)

1. Vasculitis e.g.
   Wegener's granulomatosis
   Churg–Strauss syndrome
   Microscopic polyangiitis
2. Goodpasture syndrome
3. Carcinoma of the bronchus
   (associated with membranous glomerulonephritis)
4. Legionnaire's disease
5. Renal vein thrombosis complicated by PE
   (RV thrombosis can cause haematuria in its own right, but is also associated with membranous glomerulonephritis. There is an increased risk of pulmonary embolus in RV thrombosis)

RESPIRATORY MEDICINE

7.8

a) Inadequate effort during forced expiration.

b) Give further instruction to the subject and then get her to repeat the test.

The flow volume loop shows a step in the upward portion of the expiratory curve. This part of the curve is considerably effort-dependent and abnormality in this area is often the result of lack of adequate effort during forced expiration.

Another abnormality that may be seen because of lack of effort on the part of the subject is shown in Fig. 7.11.

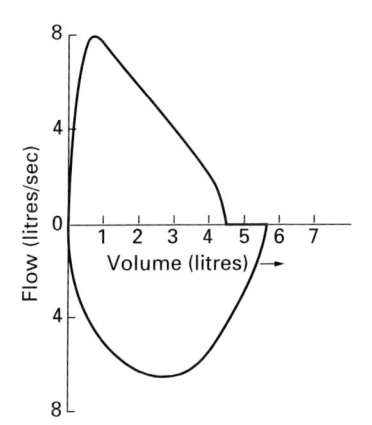

Fig. 7.11 Typical flow volume pattern produced when the subject has not taken a maximal inspiration

7.9

a) The lung function tests show a restrictive ventilatory defect together with a raised KCO and reduced T_LCO.

b) The causes of a raised KCO with reduced T_LCO are shown in Box 7.3. Conditions 2–4 are the only ones that produce a restrictive defect as well but in this case neuromuscular weakness is the most likely diagnosis since the presence of an elevated KCO makes interstitial lung disease unlikely. Although a skeletal deformity such as scoliosis, which often begins in childhood/adolescence, will produce similar lung function results it does not really qualify as a childhood illness. Diaphragmatic weakness is characterized by a low FVC that falls by a further 25% on lying flat.

c) Polio. Slowly progressive muscle weakness may occur 10–20 years after paralytic polio. This is called the 'post-polio syndrome'. The weakness is lower motor neurone in origin and affects those muscles that were initially affected by the disease. Clinically it may resemble motor neurone disease, but progression is less rapid and there are no upper motor neurone features.

Box 7.3 Causes of increased KCO with a normal or reduced T_LCO

1. Lobectomy/pneumonectomy
   (If the FVC, FEV_1, TLC and V_A are all ≈ 50% of the expected value then the patient has had a pneumonectomy: left pneumonectomy if slightly > 50%; right pneumonectomy if slightly < 50%, since the right lung is bigger than the left)
2. Neuromuscular weakness
3. Skeletal deformity e.g. scoliosis
4. Ankylosis e.g. ankylosing spondylitis
5. Pleural thickening

*Conditions 2–5 all cause a restrictive defect but, unlike the other causes of restrictive defect, the alveolar membranes are normal and gas exchange per unit volume of alveolus (i.e. KCO) is therefore unimpaired.

7.10

a) A tracheal stricture has developed as a complication of prolonged tracheostomy/intubation.

The flow volume loop shows reduction of both inspiratory and expiratory flow rates. This is the characteristic pattern of a fixed extrathoracic airway obstruction and contrasts with that of an intrathoracic large airway obstruction (that is, trachea or main bronchus), which generally shows a normal inspiratory phase with reduced flow rates in expiration when the airways tend to collapse (Fig. 7.12). The commonest cause of the latter condition is probably obstruction of a major airway by bronchogenic carcinoma.

RESPIRATORY MEDICINE

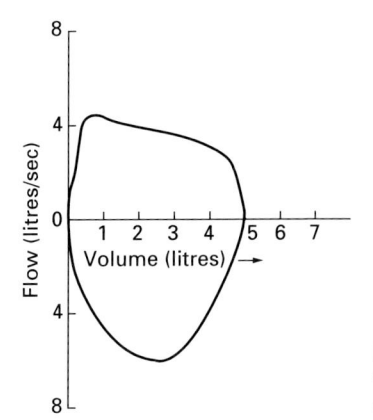

Fig. 7.12 Typical flow volume loop seen with an intrathoracic large airway obstruction

7.11

a) Multiple pulmonary emboli.

b) Multiple pulmonary arteriovenous malformations or anaemia.

The lung function tests show reduced gas transfer with otherwise normal lung function – this is a classic pattern of abnormality for the MRCP exam. Reduced gas transfer can be caused by disease affecting the integrity of the alveolar capillary membrane, ventilation perfusion mismatch or disease affecting the blood's ability to transport oxygen. Normal lung function means that lung disease is very unlikely, therefore this pattern abnormality can only be because of a problem with perfusion (multiple pulmonary emboli or multiple pulmonary AV malformations) or a problem with the blood (anaemia, methaemaglobinaemia and certain haemaglobinopathies all affect the blood's ability to transport oxygen). In this case the short history and current use of the oral contraceptive pill make multiple pulmonary emboli the most likely diagnosis.

7.12

a) Emphysema.

b) Serum protein electrophoresis to assess α_1-antitrypsin levels.

The flow rate falls off quickly during expiration because of airways collapse. This manifests as a reduction in the MEF_{50} and consequent concave deformation of the downward portion of the expiratory curve. These changes are characteristic of all forms of obstructive airways disease but are generally more marked in emphysema since airways collapse is a prominent feature of this condition and tends to occur earlier in expiration than is seen with asthma or chronic bronchitis.

This patient has developed emphysema at a very young age and this should always raise the suspicion of α_1-antitrypsin deficiency, especially in a non-smoker. The elevated liver enzymes are also compatible with this diagnosis since certain phenotypes of α_1-antitrypsin deficiency result in liver damage, which may lead to cirrhosis. If α_1-antitrypsin deficiency is found, then the patient will need genetic counselling (since it is an autosomal recessive condition) and other family members will need to be screened. The chance of developing emphysema in this condition is magnified many times if the affected individual smokes and anti-smoking advice is therefore extremely important. The risk of cirrhosis means that alcohol should only be consumed in moderation.

7.13

a) Asthma (obstructive ventilatory defect with normal or slightly increased gas transfer).

Cough and wheeze are the characteristic symptoms of asthma, but either symptom can be the predominant feature. Slightly increased gas transfer values can occur in mild asthma as a result of the fact that 1) the alveoli are normal (as distinct from chronic bronchitis and emphysema where alveoli are damaged); 2) asthmatics tend to hyperventilate; and 3) carbon monoxide (which is used to measure gas transfer) diffuses more readily across the alveolar membranes than oxygen and is therefore affected less by the obstructive defect.

8 GASTROENTEROLOGY

MALABSORPTION

Box 8.1 Main causes of generalized malabsorption	
Intestinal	
1. ↓ Surface area for absorption	
a) Villous atrophy	Coeliac disease
	Dermatitis herpetiformis
	Tropical sprue
	Giardia
b) Surgical resection	
c) Infiltration/inflammation	Crohn's disease
	Lymphoma
	Amyloidosis
	Eosinophilic gastroenteritis
	TB
	Whipple's disease
	Systemic sclerosis
d) Radiation enteritis	
2. Lymphangiectasia (lymphatic obstruction)	
a) Congenital	
b) Acquired	Lymphoma
	Constrictive pericarditis
	TB
3. ↑ Rate of transit	Carcinoid
	Thyrotoxicosis (rarely)
Pancreatic insufficiency	Chronic pancreatitis
	Pancreatic carcinoma
	Cystic fibrosis
	Pancreatectomy
	Zollinger–Ellison syndrome (excess gastric acid inactivates pancreatic enzymes)
Bile-salt mediated	Biliary obstruction
	Severe parenchymal liver disease
	Disease of terminal ileum (e.g. Crohn's)
	Terminal ileum resection
	Drugs e.g. bile acid sequestrants, neomycin, methyldopa, methotrexate, metformin, colchicine
Bacterial overgrowth	Blind loops
	Intestinal fistulae
	Intestinal diverticulae
	Intestinal strictures
	Systemic sclerosis
	Diabetes mellitus
	Hypogammaglobulinaemia
Other	Mesenteric arterial insufficiency
	Hypothyroidism

GASTROENTEROLOGY

Malabsorption is a vast disease area and encompasses malabsorption of individual constituents of the diet (e.g. Addisonian pernicious anaemia in which vitamin B_{12} malabsorption occurs in isolation) as well as generalized malabsorption. Even in this latter category there are many causes. However, malabsorption can be broadly divided into intestinal malabsorption (abnormal intestinal function); pancreatic malabsorption (abnormality of pancreatic enzyme production or secretion); bile-salt mediated malabsorption (inadequate bile salts for emulsification of fats); bacterial overgrowth; and 'other' (Box 8.1). The common causes lie within the first four categories.

8.1

See also questions 2.22, 2.23, 4.17 and 4.18

a) Malabsorption of vitamin D.

   Vitamin D is a fat-soluble vitamin and is therefore poorly absorbed if fat malabsorption occurs. Vitamin D is required for adequate absorption of calcium from the gut.

b) Secondary hyperparathyroidism.

c) Chronic pancreatitis with malabsorption of fats. Carcinoma of the pancreas is an equally acceptable answer but this usually produces chronic rather than intermittent pain. Chronic pancreatitis can also produce chronic pain, sometimes with intermittent exacerbations.

d) Alcoholism is suggested by high MCV (with normal B_{12} and folate) and high gamma GT.

   The high faecal fat indicates malabsorption, the causes of which are shown in Box 8.1 in the introductory notes to this section. Intestinal malabsorption or bacterial overgrowth would be expected to cause B_{12} or folate deficiency, and since the bilirubin is normal, significant biliary obstruction is unlikely (the liver enzymes are elevated as a result of alcohol consumption in this patient). Pancreatic insufficiency therefore remains the most likely cause; the history of recurrent abdominal pain suggests that chronic pancreatitis is the probable cause.

8.2

a) This is a normal test and it demonstrates that intestinal integrity is intact. An intestinal cause for the malabsorption is thus unlikely.

b) Cystic fibrosis.

c) Sweat sodium test: a sodium concentration of over 60 mmol/L is diagnostic of CF.

d) Further tests should aim to clarify the cause of the malabsorption and look for other complications of CF. Pancreatic function tests, liver function (hepatic cirrhosis can occur in CF), CXR and lung function tests are all indicated. Additional tests should include a glucose tolerance test since diabetes can complicate pancreatic failure.

e) Genetic counselling for parents, and for the patient when older.

The high faecal fat indicates malabsorption and, with normal intestinal integrity, failure of pancreatic exocrine function, bacterial overgrowth or failure of adequate bile salt secretion remain as the main possible causes of malabsorption (see Box 8.1). Chronic chest symptoms together with malabsorption in a child are highly suggestive of cystic fibrosis. In this condition there is abnormal chloride transport, which results in thick, viscous secretions that block glands and ducts. In the pancreas this causes chronic pancreatic insufficiency. In the lungs tenacious mucosal secretions are difficult to expectorate resulting in recurrent infections, bronchiectasis and eventual respiratory failure. Malabsorption is caused by pancreatic insufficiency. CF is caused by a mutation in the cystic fibrosis transmembrane conductance regulator gene (CTRF) on chromosome 7 and is inherited in an autosomal recessive fashion. A genetic test to assess carrier status, or whether a fetus is affected, is now available.

D-xylose absorption test

Xylose is a synthetic sugar which is absorbed unchanged from the small intestine (its absorption does not depend upon the action of enzymes) and is excreted entirely by the kidney. Thus urinary xylose excretion (and blood xylose level) following an oral dose reflects small intestinal integrity.

In a normal test, at least 23% of the oral dose is absorbed (and excreted in the urine) within the first five hours, and at least 50% of this should be within the first two hours.

False positive results can occur because of renal disease, incomplete urine collection, delayed gastric emptying and xylose-induced osmotic diarrhoea.

8.3

a) The macrocytic anaemia may represent B_{12} and/or folate deficiency. There is also fat malabsorption. There are several possible causes of this combination but in this patient one needs to exclude coeliac disease and Crohn's disease (since these are relatively common), and *Giardia* infestation (may have been contracted in Bosnia). In view of his past history of gastric ulcer surgery (this may have involved a gastroenterostomy, which can create a blind loop) bacterial overgrowth should also be excluded (bacteria metabolize dietary vitamin B_{12} thereby causing B_{12} deficiency, and also deconjugate bile salts, thereby producing fat malabsorption and steatorrhoea). The history of residence in the tropics means that one should also consider tropical sprue. This condition is endemic in the tropics (parts of Asia, some Caribbean islands, parts of South America) and consists of chronic diarrhoea with malabsorption of two or more substances (usually including B_{12} and fat). It may occur acutely or many years after the sufferer was in the tropics. Diagnosis is by exclusion of other causes of malabsorption, in conjunction with travel history. Jejunal biopsy usually shows a degree of villous atrophy, though not as severe as that seen in coeliac disease. The aetiologic agent is unknown but is presumed to be infective as it responds to treatment with antibiotics: tetracycline (together with folate supplements) is usually given, and it may be necessary to treat for up to six months.

b) Investigations should include:

- Small bowel aspirate for *Giardia* trophozoites and biopsy to show subtotal villous atrophy.
- Stool microscopy for *Giardia* cysts, and culture to exclude other enteropathogens.
- Anti-gliadin, anti-reticulin and anti-endomysium autoantibodies (for coeliac disease); anti-endomysium antibodies are the most specific.

- Small bowel meal to exclude Crohn's disease.
- Radiolabelled glycocholic acid breath test to exclude bacterial overgrowth.
- Serum B_{12} and red cell folate.

8.4

a) Gluten-sensitive enteropathy (coeliac disease).

Low calcium with low phosphate (caused by secondary hyperparathyroidism) strongly suggests either malabsorption or dietary deficiency of vitamin D (± calcium). Taken together with the macrocytic anaemia (suggestive of B_{12} or folate deficiency) and low ferritin, the clinical picture suggests malabsorption. The bilirubin is high as a result of megaloblastic anaemia, and not liver disease. Alkaline phosphatase is high because of osteomalacia. Gluten-sensitive enteropathy is suggested as a cause for the malabsorption by the presence of splenic atrophy (Howell–Jolly bodies on the blood film) and by the presence of a dimorphic blood film, which implies combined folate and iron deficiency.

b) The following tests are indicated:

- Small bowel aspirate (for *Giardia* cysts) and jejunal biopsy (to show subtotal villous atrophy).
- Anti-gliadin, anti-reticulin and anti-endomysium autoantibodies (for coeliac disease): anti-endomysium antibodies are the most specific.
- Small bowel meal to exclude Crohn's disease (and intestinal lymphoma which may be associated with coeliac disease).
- Red cell folate and serum B_{12}.

c) Folate deficiency together with iron deficiency and splenic atrophy.

A high RDW is indicative of a dimorphic (macrocytes and microcytes present) distribution of the MCV. In the context of the rest of the clinical picture the macrocytosis is likely to be caused by folate deficiency (B_{12} deficiency is unusual in coeliac disease). Target cells and microcytes (implied from the high RDW) are caused by iron deficiency (note the low

GASTROENTEROLOGY

serum ferritin) and Howell–Jolly bodies result from splenic atrophy, which is associated with gluten-sensitive enteropathy.

d) Dermatitis herpetiformis is often associated with gluten-sensitive enteropathy.

e) A gluten-free diet will improve both the malabsorption and the dermatitis herpetiformis.

Coeliac disease is caused by intolerance to the alcohol-soluble fractions of the prolamines of wheat, barley and rye. In the case of wheat, this fraction is the α gliadin component of gluten. This insensitivity results in subtotal villous atrophy of the small intestine and consequent malabsorption. The proximal small intestine tends to be more severely affected than the distal part in coeliac disease and therefore folate deficiency is almost invariable (absorbed in the duodenum), iron deficiency is common (absorbed in the jejunum and duodenum) but B_{12} deficiency is unusual (absorbed in the terminal ileum). Presentation is usually with anaemia or vague abdominal symptoms such as pain and bloating. Mouth ulcers are also common. Coeliac may be asymptomatic in up to one-third of cases though. A gluten-free diet should result in complete histological resolution (although this may take many months). Failure of resolution is caused by non-compliance with diet or incorrect diagnosis.

8.5

a) Dietary deficiency of vitamin B_{12} and vitamin D (together with inadequate sunlight exposure) in a vegan.

b) Osteomalacia resulting from vitamin D deficiency. There may also be an osteoporotic crush fracture.

c) Proximal myopathy associated with osteomalacia.

The major dietary sources of vitamin B_{12} and vitamin D are meat and dairy products. Under normal conditions dietary vitamin D is unimportant since more than required is synthesized by the skin under the action of sunlight. Dietary vitamin D becomes important in those who are housebound and in those who keep most of their body covered for religious or other reasons. Some Asian women fall into this latter category and, in addition, are vegan for religious reasons. They are therefore particularly susceptible to deficiency of these vitamins.

The macrocytic anaemia could result from B_{12} or folate deficiency but taken in this clinical context the former is more likely. Vitamin D deficiency (osteomalacia) is indicated by low calcium together with low phosphate and a raised alkaline phosphatase (see Table 2.12). The presence of normal faecal fat excretion makes malabsorption unlikely (vitamin D is a fat-soluble vitamin); therefore dietary deficiency must be the cause.

8.6

a) The presence of bacterial overgrowth is indicated by an early rise in the glycocholate breath test, and an abnormal Schilling test performed in the presence of exogenous intrinsic factor. Interpretation of the glycocholate breath test and Schilling test are described below.

b) Small intestinal diverticulae or stricture, systemic sclerosis, and 'blind loop' syndrome as a result of intestinal fistulae or previous intestinal surgery, all predispose to bacterial overgrowth.

c) The Schilling test, before and after antibiotic treatment (to kill the overgrowth), will show normalization of the test after a course of antibiotics.

[^{14}C]-glycocholic acid breath test

This measures the amount of $^{14}CO_2$ in expired air after an oral dose of [^{14}C]-glycocholic acid (a radiolabelled bile salt). Bacteria deconjugate the bile salts releasing [^{14}C]-glycine, which is metabolized to $^{14}CO_2$, and this appears in the breath. An early rise in the breath radioactivity indicates either bacterial overgrowth in the upper small intestine, or rapid transit to the colon.

GASTROENTEROLOGY

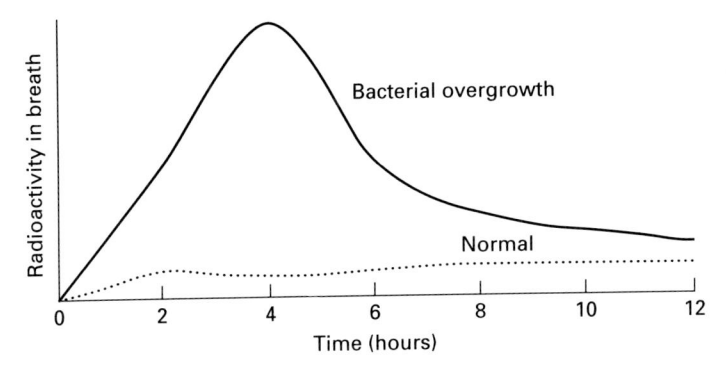

Fig. 8.1 Normal and abnormal [^{14}C]-glycocholic acid breath test results

An alternative is the hydrogen breath test in which oral lactulose is degraded by bacteria with the production of hydrogen which is measured in the expired air. An early rise in the breath hydrogen indicates bacterial overgrowth or rapid GI transit time.

Schilling test

This is used to determine the cause of vitamin B_{12} deficiency.

Part 1: 1 µg of [^{58}Co]-B_{12} is given orally to fasting patient and at the same time 100 µg of non-radioactive B_{12} is given i.m. to saturate B_{12} binding proteins and flush out the radioactive [^{58}Co]-B_{12}. All urine is then collected for the next 24 h.

Normal subjects excrete more than 10% of the radioactive dose in the urine over 24 h.

Part 2: If part 1 is abnormal then it is repeated after giving oral intrinsic factor capsules. This is part 2 of the test.

If part 2 is normal the diagnosis is pernicious anaemia.

An abnormal result for part 2 indicates either a lesion in the terminal ileum, for example Crohn's disease, or bacterial overgrowth.

Part 3: Part 2 is repeated after a course of antibiotics. If the result is now normal then the diagnosis is bacterial overgrowth; if abnormal then the diagnosis is that of a lesion in the terminal ileum.

False positive results will occur if urine collection is incomplete!

271

8.7

a) Gilbert syndrome.

b) Measure unconjugated bilirubin levels after a 16-h fast (free fatty acids released during fasting compete with bilirubin for excretion at the liver causing a further rise in the unconjugated bilirubin) and after phenobarbitone 60 mg t.d.s (phenobarbitone reduces unconjugated bilirubin to normal levels).

This patient has an elevated plasma bilirubin and the negative urine dipstick test for bilirubin means that it is the unconjugated fraction of bilirubin that is raised (conjugated bilirubin is water-soluble and can therefore travel freely in the plasma thereby allowing filtration at the kidneys; in contrast, unconjugated bilirubin is insoluble in water and therefore must travel bound to plasma proteins, which prevents excretion at the kidneys). An elevated unconjugated bilirubin level with normal liver enzymes is characteristic of Gilbert syndrome. Haemolysis can also result in increased unconjugated bilirubin with normal liver enzymes but if this were the case one would expect serum haptoglobins to be low and for a reticulocytosis to be present.

Gilbert syndrome is a benign familial disorder of conjugation and excretion of bilirubin, which results in a mildly raised unconjugated bilirubin with normal liver enzymes and a histologically normal liver. The bilirubin concentration varies considerably over time and, in most patients, the majority of the time it is not sufficiently high to cause jaundice. An increase in bilirubin levels, with consequent jaundice, may occur at times of stress such as appendicitis, as seen in this patient. The exact mode of inheritance is unclear.

Crigler–Najjar syndrome is an autosomal recessive condition in which unconjugated hyperbilirubinaemia is caused by absence (type I) or deficiency (type II) of the hepatic conjugating enzyme UDP-glucuronyl transferase. The jaundice is more severe than that in Gilbert and is present all the time.

GASTROENTEROLOGY

Box 8.2 Causes of elevated bilirubin in the absence of liver or biliary tract disease	
Conjugated	*Unconjugated*
Haemolysis*	Haemolysis*
Dubin–Johnson syndrome	Gilbert syndrome
Rotor syndrome	Crigler–Najjar syndrome (type I or type II)
	Physiological jaundice of the newborn
	Transient familial neonatal hyperbilirubinaemia
	Breast milk jaundice

*Haemolysis may cause conjugated, unconjugated or mixed hyperbilirubinaemia

8.8

a) Primary biliary cirrhosis (PBC).

b) Anti-mitochondrial antibody assay and liver ultrasound or ERCP (to exclude bile duct obstruction for example, gallstones, pancreatic carcinoma or ampullary carcinoma of bile duct) are indicated. If it had not already been performed, a liver biopsy (for histological confirmation of the diagnosis) would also be indicated.

c) The histologic features depend on the stage of the disease and are shown below. In addition, periportal cholestasis ± bile lakes may be seen. Granulomas are found in 50% of cases.

Box 8.3 Stages of primary biliary cirrhosis	
Stage	
I	Destruction of interlobular ducts
II	Ductal proliferation
III	Fibrosis
IV	Cirrhosis

This patient has biliary obstruction (elevated bilirubin with predominantly elevated alkaline phosphatase). This may be intrahepatic (blockage of intrahepatic bile canaliculi) or extrahepatic (obstruction of large extrahepatic bile ducts). However, the presence of a raised IgM together with a history of intractable pruritus suggests that primary biliary sclerosis is the diagnosis. Increased liver copper content can occur with any cause of prolonged cholestasis as well as with Wilson's disease (which may also cause liver failure). However in Wilson's disease the serum caeruloplasmin is usually low together with low serum copper and high 24-h urinary copper excretion.

PBC is a disease of unknown aetiology (thought to be autoimmune) that primarily affects middle-aged females. There is progressive destruction of the small interlobular bile ducts with fibrosis and biliary stasis. Eventually frank cirrhosis occurs. Pruritus is an early symptom and often predates the onset of jaundice. Ninety-five per cent of patients are positive for anti-mitochondrial antibody and an elevated titre of IgM is also characteristic (other immunoglobulin classes may also be elevated but not usually to the same degree as IgM).

8.9

a) Autoimmune hepatitis (autoimmune chronic active hepatitis).

This woman has hepatocellular jaundice (elevated bilirubin with predominantly elevated hepatic transaminases) and, since the liver inflammation has persisted for more than six months, chronic active hepatitis (CAH) is said to be present (by convention). The main causes of chronic active hepatitis are shown in Box 8.4, but in a female of this age, with negative hepatitis B serology, and no history of alcohol abuse or blood transfusion (suggesting hepatitis C), autoimmune chronic active hepatitis is the most likely diagnosis. Hepatitis A never becomes chronic. Polyclonal increase in immunoglobulins reflects chronic inflammation.

b) The differential diagnoses of chronic active hepatitis are shown in Box 8.4.

c) Piecemeal necrosis of periportal hepatocytes is characteristic of chronic active hepatitis. With more severe disease bridging necrosis (bridging of adjacent foci of piecemeal necrosis) is seen.

d) Investigations should be directed towards proving your primary diagnosis and excluding the other possibilities: autoimmune profile including anti-nuclear antibody and anti-smooth muscle antibody; liver ultrasound (to exclude biliary obstruction or liver infiltration/tumour); liver biopsy (to confirm chronic active hepatitis); and serology for HBV (and delta virus if HBsAg positive) and HCV are essential. Some of these tests have already been performed but additional tests include α_1-antitrypsin levels (to screen for α_1-antitrypsin

GASTROENTEROLOGY

deficiency), CXR and serum angiotensin converting enzyme (to screen for sarcoidosis) and serum copper and caeruloplasmin levels together with 24-h urinary copper excretion (to screen for Wilson's disease). Haemochromatosis would be excluded by the liver biopsy.

AIH is classified as type 1 or type 2. Classical AIH is type 1 and mainly occurs in young adult females who often have a Cushingoid appearance. Diagnosis is by exclusion of the other causes of CAH and demonstration of the presence of one or more non-organ-specific antibodies, particularly ANA and anti-smooth muscle. Immunoglobulins are characteristically greatly elevated in a polyclonal fashion (particularly IgG). Liver biopsy is essential for diagnosis. Type 2 AIH is distinguished by the presence of anti-liver/kidney autoantibodies (anti-LKM-1 antibodies). Both types may be associated with other autoimmune diseases such as Hashimoto's thyroiditis or Addison's disease.

Box 8.4 Causes of chronic active hepatitis

Alcoholism
Viral hepatitis   (HBV, HCV, δ virus in association with HBV, other non-A non-B)
Autoimmune hepatitis
Primary biliary cirrhosis
Sarcoidosis
Haemochromatosis
α_1-antitrypsin deficiency
Wilson's disease
Drugs (e.g. α-methyldopa, nitrofurantoin, isoniazid)
Cryptogenic

8.10

a) Whipple's disease.

b) Prolonged antibiotics.

The small bowel biopsy result is diagnostic for Whipple's disease. Electron microscopy would show that the macrophages are stuffed full of rod-shaped bacteria.

Whipple's disease primarily affects white males over the age of 50. It characteristically presents with diarrhoea, wasting (because of malabsorption) and arthritis but virtually any organ in the body can be involved. Affected tissues are infiltrated with foamy macrophages that are packed with the Gram-positive actinomycete, *Tropheryma wheppelii*. The diagnosis is based on demonstrating this infiltrate in biopsy specimens but PCR may be necessary to confirm this in difficult cases. Whipple's disease progresses slowly but is ultimately fatal if left untreated. Treatment is with long-term antibiotics, which must include an antibiotic that crosses the blood-brain barrier. Parenteral penicillin plus streptomycin for two weeks followed by doxycycline for one year is one recommended regime; erythromycin and cotrimoxazole have also been used. Patients generally respond well. Relapse should be treated by restarting the antibiotics or changing them if relapse occurs whilst on treatment.

8.11

a) Haemochromatosis.

b) The most useful investigations are: serum transferrin saturation (this is a more sensitive screening test than serum ferritin and will show > 80% saturation in primary haemochromatosis); serum ferritin (this is a measure of total body iron stores and it will therefore be elevated, classically to > 1000 µg/L); and liver biopsy with staining for iron (this is the gold standard and will show increased iron deposition throughout both the cellular and connective tissue components of the liver, together with cirrhosis). Other tests include a desferrioxamine excretion test (this shows elevated urinary iron excretion [> 8 mg] following desferrioxamine infusion), and, if serum transferrin saturation is not available, total iron binding capacity (TIBC will be reduced to less than 30% because of saturation of plasma transferrin by excess iron).

c) Further investigations are aimed at excluding other (possibly co-existing) causes of chronic liver disease and identifying possible complications. Appropriate tests include a glucose tolerance test to confirm diabetes; coagulation studies (impaired haemostasis may have resulted from liver disease or thrombocytopenia); liver ultrasound scan (to exclude obstructive cause of abnormal LFTs); hepatitis B/C serology; autoantibody screen (including anti-smooth muscle and anti-mitochondrial antibody); pituitary function tests; and echocardiography.

d) Impotence may be secondary to hypogonadism (as a result of pituitary dysfunction) or erectile failure (because of diabetic autonomic neuropathy and/or vascular disease.)

Idiopathic haemochromatosis is an autosomal dominant condition in which excess iron is absorbed from the bowel and deposited in various organs causing fibrosis and eventual organ failure. The liver (causing cirrhosis), endocrine glands (particularly the pancreas and pituitary causing diabetes mellitus and hypogonadotrophic hypogonadism respectively) and the heart (causing heart failure and arrhythmias) are most severely affected. The classical triad (seen in this case) of bronze skin pigmentation, hepatomegaly and diabetes mellitus (bronze diabetes) is only seen in cases of gross iron overload. Pseudogout is common through deposition of calcium pyrophosphate in both large and small joints, and it seems to particularly affect the 2nd and 3rd metacarpophalangeal joints. Treatment is with regular venesection or with desferrioxamine if venesection is not tolerated. Screening of other family members by measuring serum transferrin saturation and serum ferritin is important. Two mutations in the gene HFE on chromosome 6 have been identified and about 90% of cases of primary haemochromatosis are homozygous for one of these, most commonly (~85%) C282Y. Therefore family members suspected of having the disease should ideally have this confirmed by genetic testing since this will have implications for their own future families.

INDEX

A

Abdominal bloating 96, 268
Acetazolamide toxicity 63, 213
Acid-base balance 207–14
  disturbances 207–8
Acids, within the body 207
Acoustic trauma 80, 246
Acromegaly 170
ACTH 136, 137–41
  ectopic production 141–2
  levels 144
Addison's disease 27, 142–3, 275
Adrenal adenoma 160
Adrenal carcinoma 26, 142
Adrenal failure 27, 142–3
  causes 144
Adrenal hyperplasia 160
  congenital 32, 161
Adrenal insufficiency, secondary 27, 145–6
Alcohol, in fasting hypoglycaemia 169
Alcoholism 60, 61, 94, 191, 192, 210, 211, 265, 275
  chronic 58, 207
Alpha 1-antitrypsin deficiency 92, 99, 262, 274–5
Amenorrhoea 26, 142
  causes 154
Amiodarone 110, 117, 150
Anaemia 91, 261
  haemolytic *see* Haemolytic anaemia
  macrocytic 95, 96, 97, 267, 268, 270–1
  pernicious 97, 240, 271
  sideroblastic 48, 191
ANCA *see* Antibody, anti–neutrophil cytoplasmic
Anion gap loss, causes 209
Ankles, swollen 52, 196
Ankylosing spondylitis 87, 229, 255
Antibody, anti–neutrophil cytoplasmic 217
Aortic arch aneurysm, causes 224
Aortic arch syndrome 224
Aortic stenosis 3, 104
Appendicitis 98, 272
Arthritis 99, 275–6
  enteropathic 229
  juvenile 70, 232–3
  diagnosis 232
  psoriatic 229
  reactive 229
  seronegative causes 229
Arthropathies, crystal 230–1
Aspirin 133
Asthma 92, 253, 254, 262
  lung function abnormalities 250
Atrial fibrillation, causes 111
Atrial flutter, causes 111
Atrial septal defect 3, 103
Audiogram, normal 245
Audiology 245–8
Autoantibodies 95, 96, 267, 268
  in rheumatic diseases 216
Autoimmune haemolytic anaemia 39, 176
Autoimmune hepatitis 99, 274–5
Autoimmune thyroiditis 150
Azathioprine 187

B

Babinski sign 73
Back pain, low 97, 269–70
Bacteria, overgrowth 95, 97, 267, 270–1
Bartter syndrome 31, 158
Benzylpenicillin 235
Bilirubin
  causes of elevation 98, 273
  elevated 98, 272
Blackouts 3, 10, 14–15, 35, 168
Blalock-Taussig shunt 107
Bleeding, excessive 42, 181
Blind loop syndrome 97, 270
Bone marrow aplasia 185
Brain MRI scan 239
Brainstem, CT/MRI scan 82, 247
Breathing difficulty 90, 259–60
Breathlessness 11, 25, 40, 63, 87, 90, 91, 177, 213, 256, 259, 261
Bronchial carcinoma 19, 136, 258
Bronze diabetes *see* Haemochromatosis
Burger's disease 53, 198–9

C

Cahart's notches 248
Calcium metabolism 163–8
Candidiasis, oral 69, 227

279

Capropril challenge test 203
Carcinoid syndrome 35, 170
Cardiac arrest 16–17
Cardiac catheter studies 3–6
Cardiac hypertrophy 113
Cardiology 3–23
Cardiomyopathy
  hypertrophic 123
  hypertrophic obstructive 17, 122, 123
Carney syndrome 137
Carpal tunnel syndrome 78, 244
Cerebral abscess 73, 75, 236, 238–9
Cerebral infarction 237
Cerebrospinal fluid
  causes of elevated protein 240
  interpretation 235
Chest infections 42, 94, 180, 266
Chest pain 40, 86, 123, 177, 254
Christmas disease 182
Chronic obstructive pulmonary disease 254
Churg–Strauss syndrome 89, 216, 218, 219, 257–8
Cirrhosis 199
  primary biliary 98, 210, 273–4, 275
Coagulation disorders 180, 182
Coeliac disease 95, 96, 199, 267, 268–9
Cold agglutinins, causes 176
Collapse 14, 115
Conn syndrome 160
Connective tissue diseases 196, 224–7
Coombs' test 189
Corticotrophin releasing factor test 139
Cough
  chronic 92, 262
  dry 87, 255
  nocturnal 85, 253
CREST syndrome 68, 216, 225–6
Creutzfeld–Jakob disease 74, 238
Crigler–Najjar syndrome 98, 272–3
Crohn's disease 95, 96, 97, 218, 267, 268, 271
Cryoglobulinaemia, mixed 54, 66, 199–200, 219–20
Cullen's sign 166
Cushing syndrome 136
  causes 137
  investigation 137–41
  pituitary-dependent 25, 141
  tests interpretation 141
Cyclophosphamide 187
Cystic fibrosis 94, 266

D

D-xylose absorption test 94, 266–7
De Quervain syndrome 29, 151–2
Deafness
  bilateral conductive 81, 247
  sensorineural 79, 246
Dermatitis herpetiformis 46, 96, 188, 269
Dermatomyositis 76, 241–2
Desferrioxamine excretion test 100, 276
Dexamethasone suppression test 25, 136, 138, 139
  high-dose 26, 141
Dextrocardia 113
Diabetes insipidus
  causes 204
  cranial 56, 204
  nephrogenic 57, 205
Diarrhoea 61, 95, 99, 212, 267, 275–6
Digoxin toxicity 112
Diplopia 65, 77, 218
  intermittent 76, 240
Disseminated intravascular coagulation 43, 47, 182, 186, 189
Diverticulae, intestinal 97, 270
Dizziness 7, 8, 35, 168
Double vision *see* Diplopia
Dubin–Johnson syndrome 273
Dyspnoea, exertional 123
Dysuria 69, 229

E

Ear wax 81, 247
Eaton–Lambert myasthenic syndrome 241
Echocardiogram 3, 6
  abnormalities 17
Echocardiography 118–22
Eisenmenger syndrome 105, 106
Electrocardiogram 7–17, 108–17
  characteristics 109
Elliptocytosis, hereditary 189
Emphysema 87, 101, 256, 262

lung function abnormalities 250
Encephalitis, herpes simplex 73, 236
Endocarditis, infective 108
Endocrinology 25–37
Enteropathy, gluten-sensitive 96, 268, 269
Epilepsy 41, 179
Epistaxis 45, 186
ERCP 98, 273
Evans syndrome 186

F

FAB classification of AML 183–4
Factor IX deficiency 43, 182
Fallot's tetralogy 107
Familial Mediterranean fever 71, 233
Fanconi syndrome 212
Felty syndrome 69, 216, 226–7
Female virilization, causes 162
Fistulae, intestinal 97, 270
Flow volume loops 251–2
Fluid balance 203–7
Fluid replacement, inadequate 53, 197
Flutter waves 111
Folate deficiency 41, 95, 96, 179, 267, 268
Forced expiratory volume (FEV) 85, 250
Friderichsen-Waterhouse syndrome 142
Fructose intolerance 169

G

Galactorrhoea 156
Galactosaemia 169
Gastroenterology 94–100, 264–77
Gastroenterostomy 95, 267
Gastro–oesophageal reflux 85, 253
Giant cell arteritis 67, 221–2
Giardia infestation 95, 267
Gilbert syndrome 98, 272–3
Glomerulonephritis 201, 220
  with low C3 201
  membraneous 52, 196–7
  membranoproliferative 54, 199–200
  mesangiocapillary 54, 199–200
  mesangioproliferative 53, 198–9
  post-infectious 199
Glucose tolerance test 100, 276

Glucose-6-phosphate dehydrogenase deficiency 48, 189–90
Glycocholic acid breath test 97, 270–1
Goitre, endemic 150
Goodpasture syndrome 67, 216, 219, 223, 258
Gottron's papules 241
Gout 70, 230
Grand-mal seizures 33, 58, 164, 206
Growth hormone 170
Guillain-Barré syndrome 88, 256–7
Gut hormones 168–70

H

Haemarthrosis 43, 182
Haematology 39–50, 176–94
Haematuria 54, 199
Haemochromatosis 99, 100, 274–5, 276–7
Haemolysis, acute 191
Haemolytic anaemia 46, 188
  autoimmune 39, 176
  microangiopathic 188
  warm antibody autoimmune 180
Haemolytic-uraemic syndrome 47, 187, 189
Haemophilia B 182
Haemoptysis 67, 222–3
Hashimoto's thyroiditis 275
Heart block 115
  trifascicular 116
Heinz bodies 188, 190
Henoch-Schönlein purpura 199, 219, 220
Hepatitis
  autoimmune chronic 99, 274–5
  chronic active 218
  viral 275
Herpes simplex encephalitis 73, 236
Hirsutism 26, 30, 142, 153
  female causes 153
Histiocytosis X 204
Honeycomb lung 56, 204
Hotspot scanning *see* Infarct-avid imaging
Howell-Jolly bodies 96, 268–9
Hughes syndrome 181
Hydrocephalus 237, 239
Hydrogen breath test 97, 271
Hyperaldosteronism 32, 159–60

causes 161
Hypercalcaemia 165–6
  causes 167
Hypergammaglobulinaemia 210
Hyperkalaemia 115
Hyperparathyroidism 94, 265
  biochemical abnormalities 163
Hyperpigmentation 143
Hyperprolactinaemia, causes 157
Hypertension 55, 202
Hyperthyroidism
  causes 147
  clinical features 147
  investigation 147–52
Hyperventilation 136, 189
Hyperviscosity syndrome 177
Hypoadrenalism, differentiation 144–5
Hypocalcaemia 33, 164
  causes 165
Hypoglycaemia 143
  autoimmune 169
  causes 169
  fasting 35, 168
Hypokalaemia 115, 136
  causes 159
Hyponatraemia 143, 207
Hypothyroidism 174
  causes 150
  clinical features 147

I

IgA nephropathy 53, 198–9
IgM, raised 98, 273–4
Immunological classification of ALL 184
Impotence 30, 100, 156, 277
Infantile cyanosis 5, 107
Infarct-avid imaging 132
Infections and membraneous glomerulonephritis 196
Infectious mononucleosis 185
Insulin stress test 137, 139, 141
Interstitial lung disease, lung function abnormalities 250
Isoniazid toxicity 191

J

Jaundice 98, 99, 272, 274–5
Jervel-Lange-Nielson syndrome 117

K

Kartagener syndrome 10, 113
Karyotyping 155
Keratoconjunctivitis sicca 226–7
Kussmaul's sign 127

L

Lead poisoning 50, 194
Leg weakness 25, 136
Legionnaire's disease 223, 258
Leukaemia
  acute, cytochemical test results 183
  acute lymphocytic 183–4
  acute monoblastic 183–4
    FAB classification 183–4
  chronic lymphocytic 42, 180
  hairy cell 183
  promyelocytic acute myeloid 45, 186
Liver, increased copper content 98, 273
Lown–Ganong–Levine syndrome 109, 110
Lumbar puncture 235
Lung function tests 250–3
  abnormalities 250
Lung transfer coefficient 252
Lung transfer factor 252
Lung volumes 251
Lupus anticoagulant 180
Lupus nephritis 54, 199, 200, 201
Lymphadenopathy, cervical 44, 184
Lymphoma, intestinal 96, 268

M

McCune–Albright syndrome 137
Macrocytic anaemia 95, 96, 97, 267, 268, 270–1
Malabsorption 95, 96, 99, 165, 265, 267, 268, 275–6
  causes 264
Maladie de Roger 105
Malaria prophylaxis 48, 190
Mechanical ventilation 91, 256, 260
Megaloblastic anaemia 41, 179
Menière's disease 79, 246
Meningioma 82, 247
Meningitis
  bacterial 73, 75, 235, 238–9
  causes with low CSF glucose 236

cryptococcal 237
tuberculous 74, 237
Metabolic acidosis 60, 210
  high anion gap 59, 208, 209
  normal anion gap 208–9
Methacholine bronchial challenge test 253
Metyrapone suppression test 139–40
  results 140
Middle ear infection 239
Mineralocorticoid axis 158–63
Mitral stenosis 4, 8, 106, 124
Mitral valve leaflet, systolic anterior motion 122
Monospot test, false positive, causes 184
Moschkovitz syndrome 46, 187
Mouth ulcers 96, 269
MRI scan 239
Multiple endocrine neoplasia 36, 170–1
  endocrine involvement 172
Multiple myeloma 177, 201
  biochemical abnormalities 163
Multiple sclerosis, diagnosis 243–4
Muscle weakness 76, 241–2
  causes 242
Myasthenia gravis 76, 240–1
Mycoplasma pneumoniae chest infection 58, 206
Myelopathy 237
Myocardial infarction 21, 22, 130, 133
Myocardial perfusion scanning 131–2
Myoclonus 74, 238
Myopathy 97, 136, 269–70
Myxoma, left atrial 20, 127–9

N

Nephritis 198–9
  interstitial 200
  lupus 54, 200, 201
Nephropathy
  HIV 199
  IgA 53, 198–9
Nephrotic syndrome 52, 196
  causes 197
Nerve conduction studies 79, 244–5
Nesidioblastosis 169
Neurology 73–83, 235–48
Neuroma, acoustic 82, 247

Neuropathy, axonal sensory peripheral 244–5
Neurophysiology 240–8

O

Oedema, peripheral 19, 35, 125, 170
Oesophageal pH monitoring 253
Oral glucose tolerance test 32, 36, 170
  interpretation 171
Orthopnoea 4
Osteomalacia 96, 97, 179, 211, 268, 269–70
  biochemical abnormalities 163
Osteoporosis 136
  biochemical abnormalities 163
Otosclerosis 83, 248
Ovarian failure 30, 155

P

Paget's disease, biochemical abnormalities 163
Palpitations 5, 123
Pancreatic fistula 212
Pancreatitis 34, 94, 165, 265
Pancytopenia 43, 183
Panhypopituitarism 37, 173–4
Parathyroid hyperplasia 36, 172
Paroxysmal nocturnal dyspnoea 4
Parvovirus infection 44, 185
Patent ductus arteriosus 6, 108
Paul–Bunnell test 44, 184–5
Peak expiratory flow rate 253
Penicillamine toxicity 241
Pericardial effusion 125
  causes 127
Pericarditis, causes 127
Periodic disease *see* Familial Mediterranean fever
Pernicious anaemia 97, 240, 271
Phaeochromocytoma 173
Phenytoin toxicity 179
Pituitary adenoma 142
Pituitary disease 150
Pituitary tumour 29, 152, 156
Pituitary-adrenal axis 136–46
Pituitary-gonadal axis 153–7
Pituitary-thyroid axis 146–52
Plantar responses 55, 239
Pneumonia 60, 210

Polio 90, 260
Polyangiitis 217, 219
Polyarteritis nodosa 66, 89, 220–1, 257
Polycystic ovary syndrome 30, 153
Polycythaemia 86, 254
 causes 178
Polycythaemia rubra vera 40, 177
Polydipsia 56, 203, 204–5
 psychogenic 57, 205
Polyglandular deficiency syndrome 174
Polymyalgia, causes 222
Polymyositis 136, 241–2
Polyserositis, recurrent 71, 233
Polyuria 56, 57, 203, 204–5, 205
Porphyria, acute intermittent 49, 192
Porphyria cutanea tarda 49, 192, 193
Porphyrias 193
Post-nasal drip 85, 253
Post-polio syndrome 90, 260
Precocious puberty, causes 162
Pregnancy test 28, 151
Primary sclerosing cholangitis 218
Probenecid 190
Procainamide 110
Prostatic cancer 43, 182
Proteinuria 54, 200
Pruritis 98, 273–4
Pseudogout 100, 277
Pulmonary arteriovenous malformations 91, 261
Pulmonary embolus 91, 177, 254, 261
Pulmonary fibrosis 87, 255
Pulmonary hypertension 4, 5, 105, 106, 113
 causes 114
Pulmonary-renal syndrome 223
 causes 258
Pyelonephritis 205
Pyloric stenosis 61, 211
Pyrazinamide toxicity 191
Pyruvate kinase deficiency 185, 189

Q
QT interval, prolonged 117

R
Radioactive isotope scanning 140
Radionuclide imaging 131
Raynaud syndrome, causes 225
Reiter syndrome 229
 extra-articular features 230
 incomplete 69, 229–30
Renal angiography 202
Renal artery stenosis 202
Renal biopsy 200
Renal failure 13, 115
 pre- 53, 197–198
Renal medicine 52–63, 196–214
Renal stones 60, 210, 211
Renal tubular acidosis, types and causes 60, 210–11, 212, 213–14
Renal vein renin ratio 203
Renal vein thrombosis 258
Renogram, isotope 55, 202
Resistant ovary syndrome 155
Respiratory acidosis 60, 210
 compensated 59, 210
Respiratory medicine 85–92, 250–62
Restrictive ventilatory defect 87, 255
 causes 256
Reticulocytosis 190
Rheumatoid arthritis 69, 226–7
Rheumatoid factor 65, 216, 219
Rheumatology 65–71, 216–33
Rickets, vitamin D-resistant 34, 167
Riedel's thyroiditis 150
Romano-Ward syndrome 117
Romanowski staining 194

S
Sacroiliitis 255
Salicylate overdose 62, 213
Sarcoidosis 275
Schilling test 97, 270–1
Schirmer's test 226–7
Schmidt syndrome 174
Scleroderma 226
Sclerodermoid diseases 226
Sheehan syndrome 150
Sick euthyroid syndrome 28, 149
Sickle-cell disease 44, 185
Sideroblastic anaemia 48, 191
Single photon emission computerized tomography 132
Situs inversus 113
Sjögren syndrome 69, 210, 211, 226–7
 autoantibodies 216
Smoking 223
Spherocytosis, hereditary 185, 189
Spinal block 75, 239

Spinal cord compression 136
Spirometry 250
Spleen, atrophy 96, 268–9
Spondyloarthropathies 228–30
   clinical features 228
Still's disease 70, 232
Sulphonamides 188, 190
   toxicity 192
Synacthen test 27, 142, 144–5, 146
Syndrome of inappropriate ADH
   secretion 58, 74, 206, 237
   causes 206
Synovial fluid, abnormalities 231
Syphilis 201
Systemic lupus erythematosus 219
   drug-induced 202
Systemic sclerosis 97, 225–6, 270

T

Takayasu's disease 68, 223
Tensilon test 240
Thalassaemia, beta trait 41, 178
Thallium scan 131
Thrombocytopenic purpura
   immune 45, 186
   thrombotic 46, 187
Thrombosis
   deep venous 42, 180
   renal vein 196
Thymoma 241
Thyroiditis
   autoimmune 150
   congenital 150
   iatrogenic 150
   subacute 29, 151–2
Thyrotoxicosis 28, 111, 146
Thyroxine 29, 151
Thyroxine-binding globulin, altered
   levels 151
Tinnitus 79, 246
Tropical sprue 95, 267
TSH hypersecretion syndrome 29,
   152
Tuberculosis, pulmonary 48, 191
Tubular necrosis, acute 198
Tumours
   bone metastasis 166
   ectopic ACTH production 141–2
   and membraneous
      glomerulonephritis 196
Turner's sign 166

U

Ulcerative colitis 218
Ureterosigmoidostomy 212
Urinary tract infection 57, 205
Uroporphyrin 192

V

Vasculitis 200, 217–24, 220, 223, 258
   classification and causes 217
   cutaneous 220
Ventricular septal defect 4, 105
Ventricular tachycardia 115
   torsade de pointes 117
Ventricular thrombus 130
Virilization, female 162
Vision, blurred 26, 142
Visual evoked potentials 77, 242
   calculation of latency 243
Vitamin B12 deficiency 95, 96, 267,
   268
   dietary 97, 269–70, 271
Vitamin D deficiency 165, 179
   dietary 96, 97, 268, 269–70
Von Gierke's disease 169
Von Willebrand's disease 181

W

Waldenström' s macroglobulinaemia
   177
Water deprivation test 56, 203
Wegener's granulomatosis 65, 89, 217,
   218–19, 257
Weight loss 95, 96, 99, 267, 268,
   275–6
Whipple's disease 99, 229, 275–6
Wilson's disease 98, 273–4, 275
Woolf–Parkinson–White syndrome 7,
   109

Z

Zollinger–Ellison syndrome 171

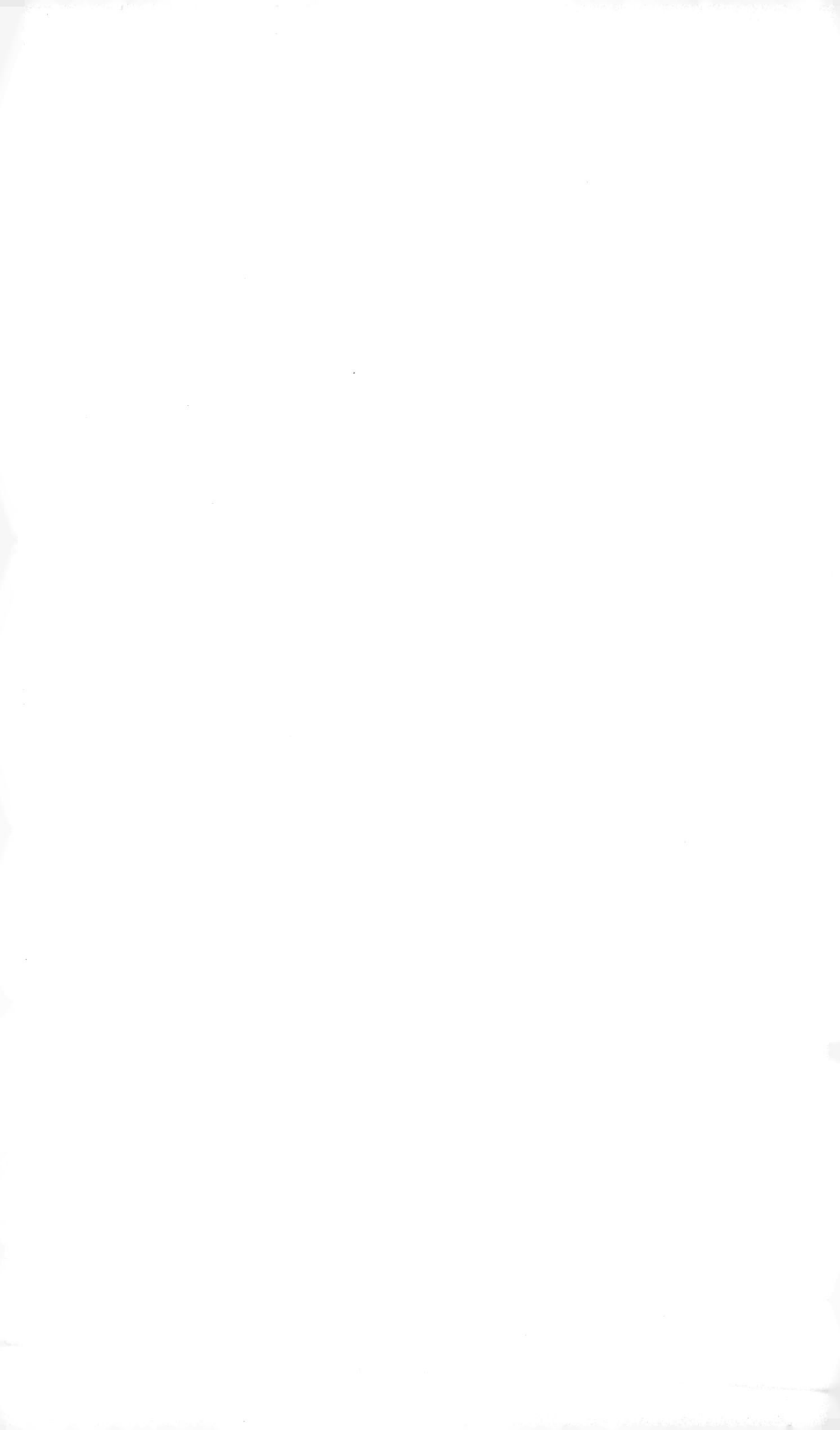

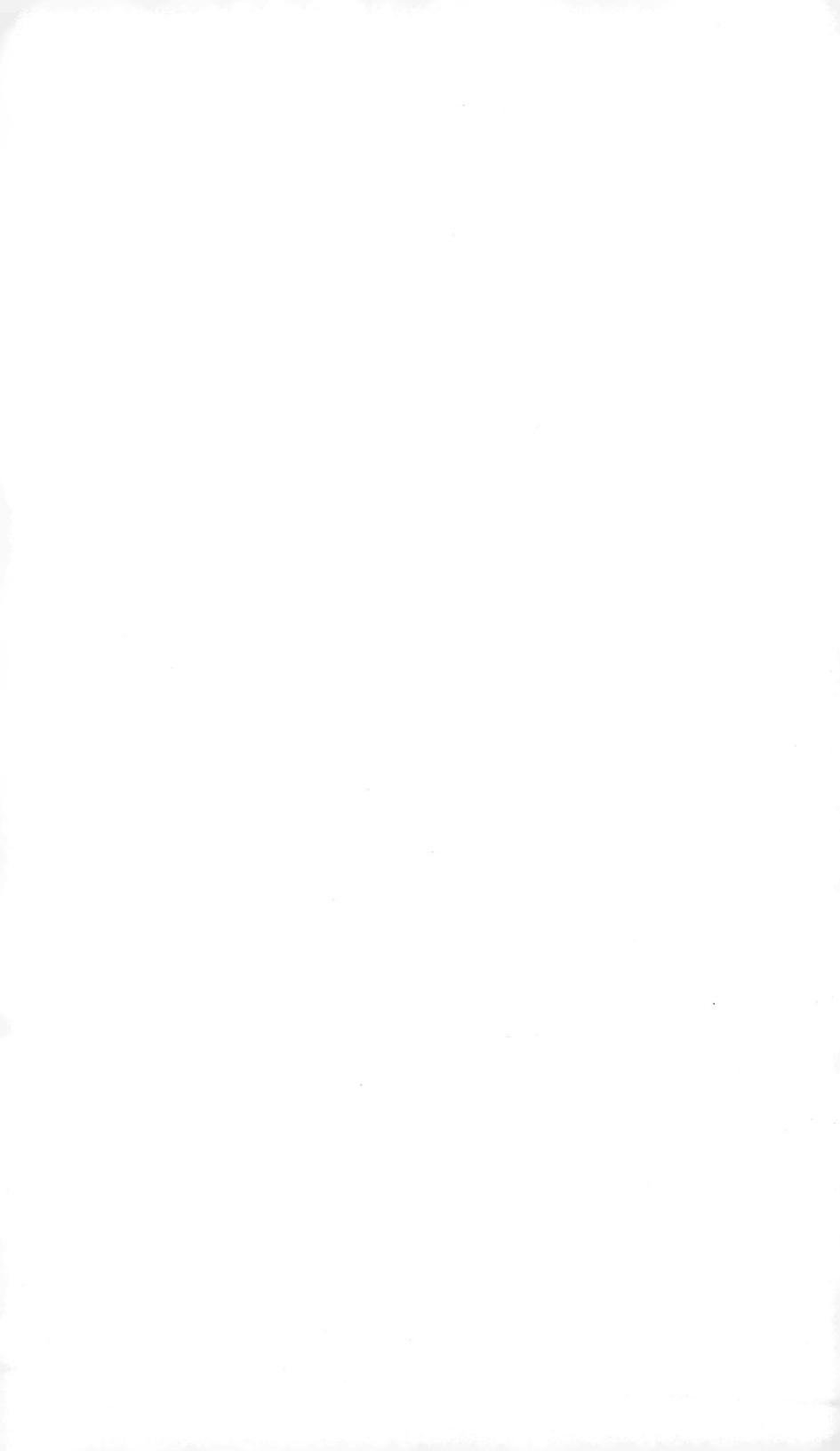